U0701961

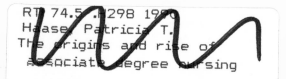
DATE DUE

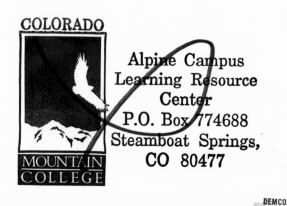

The project which made this book possible

was funded by the W. K. Kellogg Foundation

of Battle Creek, Michigan.

The Origins and Rise of

Associate Degree Nursing Education

Patricia T. Haase

Companion Volume to *Associate Degree Nursing Education:*

An Historical Annotated Bibliography, 1942–1988

The National League for Nursing

Duke University Press   Durham and London 1990

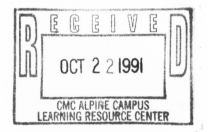

© 1990 Duke University Press
All rights reserved
Printed in the United States of America
on acid-free paper ∞
Library of Congress Cataloging-in-Publication Data
Haase, Patricia T.
The origins and rise of associate degree nursing education /
Patricia T. Haase.
Companion vol. to: Associate degree nursing education : an
historical annotated bibliography, 1942–1988.
Includes bibliographical references.
ISBN 0-8223-0991-2.—ISBN 0-8223-0978-5 (pbk.)
1. Nursing—Study and teaching (Associate degree)—United States—
History.   I. Haase, Patricia T. Associate degree nursing
education.   II. Title.
[DNLM: 1. Education, Nursing, Associate—history—United States.
WY 11 AA1 H110]
RT74.5.H298   1990
610.73'071'73—dc20
DNLM/DLC
for Library of Congress   89-13405 CIP

For my father

Lawrence Edmond Thompson

Contents

Preface

This narrative and its companion volume, *Associate Degree Nursing Education: An Historical Annotated Bibliography, 1942–1983*, originated in the late 1970s in discussions among leaders in nursing education about the future of community college education for nurses. The educators had been assembled by the W. K. Kellogg Foundation of Battle Creek, Michigan, to review the accomplishments of Kellogg-funded projects in associate degree in nursing (ADN) education and to discuss what might be done next. (To that date, Kellogg had allocated many millions of dollars for numerous projects to encourage development of ADN programs.) Much of the discussion of future directions focused on the difficulties resulting from the existence of several types of basic nursing education. The most controversial of these were the issues of titling and licensure.

Most observers agree that the controversy surrounding basic education in nursing will continue as long as there is more than one kind of school a person may attend in order to become a nurse. The three existing programs—the two-year ADN program, the three-year diploma program, and the four-year baccalaureate program—all qualify their graduates for state examinations for licensure. But the nurse's working world does not recognize, by licensing procedures, by titles, by pay, or by work assignment, the differences between the three programs. The resulting controversies among nurse educators have troubled nursing for years, but the issues are little understood by others, even by other health professionals.

One problem that was laid bare during the meetings at the Kellogg Foundation was the widespread ignorance even among nurses and professional educators about the origins and distinctive characteristics of the ADN program, despite its recent origin and the fact that ADN pro-

grams and graduates outnumber all others. In the belief that such ignorance can only complicate a difficult situation, Kellogg officials agreed
to underwrite the costs of a dissemination project as a part of their
most recent ADN projects (described in this volume in chapters 10 and
11). The mission of the dissemination project would be to assemble the
facts about the rise of the ADN degree and to see that they were circulated to as wide a readership as possible. I was selected to direct the
project, known officially as the Dissemination Project: Print Materials
to Describe the Kellogg Projects in Associate Degree Education.

I have been convinced for many years both as a nursing program
director and as a researcher in nursing history that a clearinghouse of
information about the ADN, resembling ERIC for education generally,
needed to be established. It is my firm belief that until information
about ADN education is readily available, participants in the ongoing
debate about levels of practice will only repeat themselves endlessly,
unaware that they are discussing issues that have been examined before.
This narrative account of the rise of the ADN and its companion bibliography volume represent the first steps in the establishment of just
such a repository of information.

The ADN dissemination project was funded in 1985, and our
research began shortly thereafter. The original plan was to assemble
one document, an account of the history of the ADN degree accompa-
nied by a listing of all the sources used in writing it. The long-term
hope was that the research files of the project could form the database
of an eventual clearinghouse or on-line service. Research had not proceeded far before it became apparent that sheer bulk would make a
complete listing of the resources impossible to fit at the end of a book.
Focus then shifted to the production of two books, one an annotated
bibliography, the other a narrative.

The narrative covers that period in American history from just after
World War II to the middle of the 1980s. This period was selected so
that we could trace the roots of the ADN idea as well as its development and the conditions in health care that caused its promotion and
rapid rise to prominence.

Disagreements about the associate degree program at its inception
and thereafter, its practices and policies, are presented from the point of
view of an interested observer. Arguments for one point of view or
another are not pursued. Readers who are strongly for or against a particular issue in ADN education may feel that this narrative of events is

biased on some points, but they must rest assured that persuading readers to take a stand was not my intent.

The support of the W. K. Kellogg Foundation for ADN education has been highlighted because of the foundation's continuing commitment to the purposes of the associate degree movement. It has provided several million dollars to faculties and other groups to explore and demonstrate the ADN idea. The federal government has also been a strong financial backer of the ADN idea, and this study is the first to focus attention on the federal contribution to the movement.

Acknowledgments

The narrative, like the companion bibliography, is the product of the labors of many people, most of them specialists whose talents and perseverance have made a massive task seem almost manageable.

The project was centered in my office at the University of Tennessee at Chattanooga. Through the many months of research and writing, I have enjoyed the unfailing support and administrative ability of assistant project director Patricia L. Goodman. Part of the research and all the editorial work were conducted in Atlanta under the supervision of Dr. Barbara B. Reitt, who has similarly assisted me as a consultant on other nursing education projects. Without her help, this volume would never have been completed. She not only helped with the research, she corrected my prose, rephrased many paragraphs, and kept a sharp eye for confused and unclear sentences. I express my deep gratitude for her constant assistance. She has worked with nursing publications for many years and has an uncanny ability to ask questions that clarify the issues most decisively. No one could have been more generous or more expert in her devotion to the task.

In this project's earliest stages, research in the ADN literature was conducted at the University of Tennessee at Chattanooga by Onalee Johnson, RN. Subsequent research was directed from Atlanta by Dr. Reitt, who was assisted by Dr. Stephen J. Goldfarb, Daphna W. Gregg, RN, and Dr. Virginia Ross. Dr. Goldfarb was especially helpful in assembling in long tables nursing education statistics that are available only in widely scattered sources. His meticulous work relieved us of one of the worst worries of historical writing, that of finding just the right fact at the right time. I wish also to thank Sandra Thomas of the University of Tennessee at Chattanooga faculty for traveling with me to visit the graduate project sites. Her notes taken during the visits were valuable to me in writing the chapter that describes the projects in graduate education.

It was my pleasure to travel to each of the project sites, and I wish to express my appreciation to all the project directors and their staffs. They were generous with both time and expertise, for which I thank them. And I salute them for their courage and perseverance in completing the missions of their respective project tasks.

Several specialists in computer database searches made important contributions throughout the project. We remember with particular gratitude the proficiency and discipline of the late Irene Malleson, head of the Science Department of Woodruff Library at Emory University. We benefited also from the advice of Elizabeth McBride, head of the Documents Department at Woodruff Library, who initiated us in the arcana of the federal Depository System. We were assisted as well by Gail Christian, of the Georgia State University library system, who searched government databases for us. We are also much indebted to the able staff members in charge of the records and archives at the National League for Nursing in New York and the Kellogg Foundation in Battle Creek, who were unfailingly patient about our need to locate many items quickly during our visits to their collections.

The editorial management of the mounds of cards and computer printouts, and later of the many revisions of both the bibliography and the narrative, has been the responsibility of Marie S. Morgan, whose intelligence and discipline have made the difference between system and chaos. She has copyedited text with a fine hand and has coordinated as well the work of clerical specialists: Martha Hagan of Word Wizards has indeed performed magical feats for us with her word processing; proofreading heroism must be credited to Wendy Barringer, Adrian Fillion, Sally Godshall, Jeannie H. McCormack, and Kate Ramsey.

Early analysis to prepare for eventual indexing was done for us by Sally Godshall. All subsequent indexes for both volumes were compiled by Kimberley C. Vivier, whose precision and intelligence have saved us from many an error.

Finally, I am grateful for the advice, assistance, and counsel of early leaders in the ADN movement. Marie L. Piekarski, of the University of Kentucky Community College System, has generously lent us copies of now rare books in her collection of ADN materials. Equally generous with their resources, both printed and personal ones, have been the members of the project's Advisory Committee: Virginia Allen, Margaret Applegate, Georgeen Harriet DeChow, Mildred Montag, and Verle Waters. These people have met with us on several occasions to offer their advice and to answer our questions. They have been constantly ready, as well, to answer even the smallest questions raised during the research stages of our work. We are grateful to them not only for making their knowledge available but also for their wisdom.

Patricia T. Haase

I

The Roots of the ADN Idea

Every story in the mosaic of history has a beginning, a cast of characters, a set of social circumstances, and its own momentum. The development of a new, two-year program for educating professional nurses during the years just after World War II is no exception. The story of the associate degree in nursing (ADN) begins in the nurse shortage crisis of the late 1940s and continues in frequent controversy through the decades that followed. The ADN, so revolutionary at its inception, has weathered thirty-five stormy years and is now an established part of educational practice.

To understand why a two-year program ever came to be, one must understand the changes in health care and higher education at the end of World War II. The rapid rise of the ADN idea depended on the convergence of several urgent needs that came to the forefront of the public consciousness at this time. R. Louise McManus called the situation "fortuitous," but much more than mere chance was at work.[1] The immediate occasion for the development of the ADN program was a concern over a looming shortage of nurses. Nurses were in short supply because the demand for their services rose sharply. The postwar demand was attributable to three developments: the recent advancement of the ability of Americans to treat disease, an expansion and upgrading of hospital facilities, and the growing number of Americans enrolled in private health care insurance programs. Nursing shortages have been a chronic problem for the American health care system ever since World War II, and they figure prominently in our story. But solving a nursing shortage was not the only motive behind the development of the new degree program. A reform movement in nursing intent on moving nursing education into the general system of American higher education was also to play an important role.

What is startling, indeed unique, about the origins of the ADN program is that it took hold so quickly; only about a dozen years separate its beginnings on paper in 1948 from its solid establishment in junior and community colleges in the 1960s. It is the only degree program in American higher education not to have been the result of slow development over many years. The two-year nursing program not only caught on, it spread like wildfire. This study and the research that produced the companion volume on the literature about the associate degree are the fruits of an attempt to learn why the ADN so quickly became the dominant program in nursing education in terms of both the number of schools and the number of graduates.

War Shortages

Throughout the early 1940s the nation invested manpower and resources to help fight the war. Professional nurses contributed heavily to the war effort, both directly, in military service, and indirectly, by extending their work hours in civilian hospitals at home. More than 65,000 nurses served in the field during the war, approximately 11,000 in the navy and 54,000 in the army.[2] At home, nurses worked extended hours—averaging 48- to 60-hour work weeks—to make up for the short staffing in civilian hospitals. By 1944–1945 the student nurses being trained in the nation's 1,300 hospital-affiliated schools of nursing (at the time, the backbone of nursing education) made up fully 80 percent of the total nursing work force in the nation's hospitals. That meant, of course, that hospital nursing on the home front was largely in the hands of the incompletely trained novice working under the direction of an overworked supervisor. This was not a new pattern in the workplace; what was new was that the numbers of nurses available for civilian care were lower. Moreover, as industry tooled up for the war effort, it siphoned off yet many other nurses; 13,800 RNs were employed in industrial settings, fully twice as many as before the war.

The shortage was so acute that in 1941 New York's Mayor Fiorello H. LaGuardia, in his role as director of civilian defense, developed a nationwide program for training volunteer nurse's aides to work at the side of the registered nurse in the hospital. He invited 800 nursing schools to participate, along with the Red Cross and the Office of Civilian Defense.[3] Throughout the war, civilian hospitals relied heavily on the work of such volunteers, trained in intensive courses, to supplement the work of beleaguered nurses in hospitals. The nation's experience with the problems of training these nursing assistants and with finding ways to use them effectively in the general hospital would have important implications for nursing practice and education in later years.

The wartime strain on the nation's health care resources was immense. In 1943 a total of 170,599 nurses were trained and licensed, capable of staffing the nation's hospitals; 35,000 were serving with the military. According to one report, nearly half of the nation's active RNs volunteered for military service, but physical incapacity and the nation's civilian needs kept most at home.[4] Nonetheless, by 1944 the American Hospital Association (AHA) reported that 23 percent of the nation's hospitals were being forced to close beds, wards, and operating rooms because of the lack of nurses.[5]

But despite the apparent willingness of American nurses to serve in the war effort, near the end of the war there arose the fear that even the military was experiencing an acute nursing shortage. The concern was so great that on 6 January 1945 Roosevelt called for a nurse draft, declaring that the nation's need was "too pressing to await the outcome of further efforts at recruiting."[6] His unprecedented call for the drafting of women into military service followed close upon the heels of a column by Walter Lippmann in which he charged that wounded soldiers were being neglected because of the lack of nurses.[7] There were also reports that eleven army units had been sent into the field without a single nurse; each unit should have had eighty or ninety nurses attached. And Clare Booth Luce, at the time a member of the House Committee on Military Affairs, told the press that American women "have not been doing their part as well as the British."[8] She wondered if something might be wrong with the way the American nurses were being trained and recruited.

Committees in the House and the Senate discussed a bill to draft nurses; it passed in the House but bogged down in the Senate as the end of the war drew near. In the meantime, stung by the criticisms, American nurses responded with a "mass of applications" for commissions, 10,000 of which were filed between 8 January and 29 January 1945. In addition, an unprecedented 60 percent of the senior nursing students receiving their training at that time under auspices of the Cadet Nurse Corps chose service in the military, apparently responding to either the nation's need or the threat of a draft.[9]

The fear of a nursing shortage in the military may have been unfounded or exaggerated, a consequence of bureaucratic mismanagement, but it was certainly ill-timed. The war was coming to an end; victory in Europe came in May, and Japan surrendered in August. By the end of the year the army found too many of its 54,291 graduate nurses idle, and Colonel Florence A. Blanchfield, superintendent of the Army Nurse Corps, released 2,000 of them for civilian employment.[10]

What are we to make today of the contradictory statistics and claims about nursing shortages during and at the end of the war? Whether or not the shortage existed before the war is not possible to determine, because the statistics on nurse manpower were collected piecemeal by numerous groups, private and public, and their figures rarely jibe. Nevertheless, it is obvious that during the war the civilian side of health care suffered from genuine nursing shortages. And in any event, the nation emerged from war more conscious than ever of its need for highly trained nurses and acutely sensitive to the possibility that nursing shortages might continue to be a problem if nothing were done at the national level to prevent them.

The National Response to Shortages

National leaders in nursing responded to the threat of war in 1940, the year before Pearl Harbor, by forming the Nursing Council on National Defense. The newly elected president of National League for Nursing Education (NLNE), Isabel Stewart, suggested the formation of "some official nursing committee or commission to think through the position that nurses should take with respect to national defense and the many adjustments that may be called for within the next few months." Stewart expressed the belief that "we should have such a commission on board that is representative of the nursing profession as a whole and that it should be at work now, and not wait until [the Red Cross] . . . calls on us to do something."[11] Within weeks of Stewart's making the suggestion, recalls Stella Goostray,

> representatives of five national nursing organizations—ANA, NOPHN, NLNE, NACGN, ACSN, and representatives of several Federal agencies—Army Nurse Corps, Navy Nurse Corps, Children's Bureau, USPHS, Divisions of State Relations and of Hospitals, Nursing Service, Veterans Administration Nursing Service, Department of Indian Affairs, and the ARCNS met in New York.

By the end of that day, the Nursing Council on National Defense was on its way.[12]

Thus, even before the United States became involved in the hostilities, leaders in professional nursing began to coordinate their efforts at the national level. The council they created remained active long after the war, passing through a number of name changes. This council would profoundly affect the course of nursing history. It proposed the study of the nursing profession that became known as the Brown Report and later reconstituted itself as a committee to implement the report. The Brown Report proposed that nurses be trained in colleges and universities, not as hospital employees. The effort to bring about that change galvanized professional nursing during the late 1940s.

Not only were nurses themselves creating the structures within the profession that would play a critical role in the changes and reforms of the postwar years, but the federal government was also setting up programs, agencies, and patterns of funding that would affect postwar nursing programs.

On 1 July 1941, just seven months after Pearl Harbor, President Roosevelt signed the Labor-Federal Security Appropriation Act, which earmarked $1.8 million for nursing education. Heretofore, federal funds for nursing education had always been targeted for specialized fields, particularly public health nursing. But these funds were to be used, among other things, for refresher courses for inactive nurses and for basic schools of nursing so that they could increase the number of students they were enrolling. The U.S. Public Health Service (USPHS) would administer these funds, advised by consultants from the nursing profession. The program had widespread impact, as funds for one purpose or another were awarded to a total of 114 schools of nursing throughout the nation.[13]

As the United States became directly embroiled in the war and concern about the need for nurses grew, the pressure to increase government support for nursing education continued to build. For example, Annie W. Goodrich, the dean emeritus of the Yale University School of Nursing, argued that nursing education needed to be a part of the nation's educational system, receive governmental support, and be based on the baccalaureate degree.[14] A. C. Haupt recommended that nursing, to meet the war emergency, recruit more students into nursing schools, use aides to assist professional nurses, and distribute trained RNs more effectively.[15]

The federal support for nursing education did increase; Congress appropriated $3.5 million for that purpose for fiscal year 1942–1943, doubling its previous appropriation.[16] And the Federal Security Agency sponsored a series of conferences in which possible solutions to nursing shortages were explored. The nursing leaders and hospital administrators who deliberated at these meetings joined in backing legislation proposed in Congress in the spring of 1943 by Representative Frances Payne Bolton of Ohio. The Bolton Act, creating the United States Cadet Nurse Corps, was enacted into law on 15 June 1943. Now, for the first time in the nation's history the federal government would subsidize the entire education of a nurse, not only paying for direct educational costs but providing a monthly stipend as well. It was not necessary for the student to show financial need, only that she promise to serve in essential nursing for the duration of the war. She could choose either military or civilian service. As we have seen, except when the threat of a nurse draft loomed in 1945, the majority of the cadets chose civilian service in their home hospitals (73 percent).[17]

The Bolton Act resulted in two developments critical to nursing in the long run. First, the standard three-year nursing program was accelerated, as cadet nurses were trained in thirty months. Because state boards of nursing required thirty-six months, the cadets served six-month practice assignments before becoming eligible for licensure. Nevertheless, it was during the war and under USPHS auspices that an abbreviated curriculum for training the registered nurse was first developed and that the use of both colleges and universities by nursing schools was expanded.[18] And second, the Division of Nurse Education of the USPHS was established. It was headed initially by Lucile Petry, formerly the dean of the Cornell University–New York Hospital School of Nursing. She was advised by a committee of nurse educators appointed by the Federal Security Administrator.[19]

The wartime federal impact on nursing education was profound and far-reaching. Under the Lanham Act of 1941, $17 million in building funds were appropriated for the construction of residences and educational buildings. Nursing school enrollments increased 30 percent after 1943, thanks to the Bolton Act. By the time the program was ended in 1948, 125,000 student nurses had graduated as cadets, 15,000 had received funds for advanced study, and the government had spent a total of $160 million on aid to nursing students. In 1945 alone the federal appropriation for the Cadet Nurse Corps represented more than half of the entire USPHS budget.[20]

Advances During the War: Medical Practice

By current standards, American medicine could do all too little when the nation entered the war, for doctors had little with which to attack disease except for quinine and for salvarsan to treat syphilis. A few vaccines had been developed and were in use. Antitoxins for tetanus, rabies, and diphtheria were available, as were vitamins, insulin, liver extract, aspirin, opium, and digitalis. But the so-called miracle drugs were only just beginning to be discovered.

Today, accustomed to the ready availability of a great variety of such drugs, we little appreciate the astounding difference the new drugs made in the care of the sick and the wounded. Lewis Thomas recalled in 1980:

> These events were simply overwhelming when they occurred. I was a medical student at the time of sulfanilamide and penicillin, and I remember the earliest reaction of flat disbelief concerning these things. We had given up on therapy a century earlier. . . . We were educated to be skeptical about the treatment of disease.
>
> Overnight, we became optimists, enthusiasts. The realization that disease could be turned around by treatment was a totally new idea.[21]

In all, approximately 200 of the new miracle drugs were developed. Today, about one-fifth of all prescriptions are for antibiotics. They have revolutionized both the surgical and medical approaches to treatment; without them, few of the developments in modern medicine since World War II would have been feasible.

The revolution in surgery that occurred during the war was nearly as dramatic as the changes in medical treatment of disease. "Surgery before World War II was all big surgery," declared one surgeon. "It was difficult surgery . . . for the most part, gross surgery . . . the removal of tumors and the amputation of legs because of diabetic gangrene—things like that."[22] But once infection could be treated with antibiotics, new surgical procedures could develop rapidly, and surgical schedules grew heavy. Also, at the outbreak of the war, new anesthetizing drugs were becoming available: sodium pentothal was used, IV spinals were available, and curare-like relaxants were sometimes administered.

Not only was the treatment of patients changed during the war years, the medical profession began to change as well. In 1940 only 23.5 percent of all physicians were specialists, but a survey in 1945 revealed that 63 percent planned to specialize after the war. An article in the journal of the American Medical Association (AMA) in 1946 noted the heightened demand for advanced training: "In 1941, before the war, there were 5,256 physicians in approved . . . residencies and fellowships . . .[;] today there are 8,930, an expansion of 70 percent."[23] Physicians were heavy participants in the GI Bill (the Service Man's Readjustment Act of 1944), which provided many with the means to obtain the training for specialty practice.

The impact of all these medical changes on the nation's health care system generally and on nursing in particular was profound. More diseases were considered treatable; more, and more difficult, surgery was being performed; specialization was pushing practice into more advanced and more refined arenas. Overall, a more aggressive and optimistic mode of health care would mean, inevitably, a heightened demand on nursing: not only for more, but for more highly skilled nurses.

The Government Assumes a Role

The situation in the nation's health care system right after the war exerted great pressure on the nursing schools, which were ill equipped to respond adequately. To begin with, the civilian health care system was overwhelmingly private. Before the war the government paid only 20 percent of the nation's health bill. A distrust of government had seemed natural in a people that included so many who had come to this country to escape despotism. Each ethnic or religious group developed its own social and health services, most notably its own system of hospitals. Leading hospitals in one city after another were religiously affiliated, for example, creations of private groups, often of local constituencies. Public hospital facilities were most often associated with care of the poor and were thereby suspected of providing a lower quality of care.

Servicemen and -women came home to a different, more powerful America. The nation was now the leader of the free world, and victory in war made any goal seem accomplishable. The mood was sharply different from that of the depression years. The economy turned upward as industry began a period of energetic growth. Where their health was concerned, people wanted quality care, and the progress made during the war only increased the desire for more and better care. Yet, in 1945 health insurance was held by only a small proportion of the American people. The demand for coverage was light, a carryover of prewar attitudes; there had been so little by present standards that medicine could do to cure disease, and people commonly avoided using hospitals, fearing them and their expense.

Now, government was proposing a tax-supported health plan. Truman's Fair Deal envisioned a new role in health care for the federal government. His ideas had precedents from the Roosevelt years. In 1934, for example, the federal government enacted the Social Security Act. In 1939 Senator Robert F. Wagner of New York proposed that the states develop health insurance programs and step up existing medical services. And in 1944 Roosevelt issued the Second Bill of Rights, with the clear implication that the federal government should underwrite each person's right to a job, an education, food, and medical care. Those in need, argued the president, are not free.

But despite the heavy involvement of government in health services during the war, the majority of Americans continued to prefer private over public sponsorship of health care delivery. When President Truman proposed an ambitious program that included national health insurance, it was defeated by the many who feared a socialist-oriented health care system. The Murray-Wagner-Dingell bill, introduced in November 1945, was defeated after extensive and heated testimony during the spring of 1946. The bill included provisions for expanded public health services, for medical and nursing education, for research, for national health insurance, and for hospital construction. (The NLNE supported the bill; the American Nurses' Association [ANA] did not.) Much of this was ultimately enacted, in some form, during the following decades. But in the immediate postwar years, the resistance to such thoroughgoing government involvement was too strong for it to be enacted as a whole.

The one proposal that was quickly enacted concerned federal support of hospital construction. When it was proposed separately as the Hill-Burton bill, the opposition was much less intense and the funding was approved in 1946. (We will return to the Hill-Burton Act and its impact on nursing.)

Nurse Education After the War

The overwhelmingly private nature of the health care system explains in part the poor status of nursing education after the war. Most nurses were educated in three-year programs operated by the hospitals; each hospital, in short, produced its own nurses. Of course, not all the graduates would remain in the hospital's employ, but those who did worked with the not-insignificant assistance of the captive labor pool formed by the current crop of nursing students.

The education these students received was not like the postsecondary study pursued by students in other fields. The nurses received on-the-job training in what amounted to an apprenticeship system. They worked long and hard, 44 to 48 hours a week, in addition to their hours in the classroom. The teaching was often provided by nurses and physicians on the hospital staff rather than by faculty employed by the school. Evening and night tours of duty were the rule, not the exception. The students were usually not paid for their work on the hospital floor; instead, they paid a nominal tuition (author Haase's own tuition, for example, was $125 a year) to pay for the cost of the education, living accommodations, and uniforms.

The setting was cloistered and the work difficult. It was training in the tradition of a frontier society, and it was becoming apparent to increasing numbers of people that it was an outmoded system.[24] Nor was it successful in recruiting the larger number of new students that the expanding system demanded.[25] As the specter of a nursing shortage once again caught the public attention, the focus was on the nursing school.

The Nursing Shortage Becomes Chronic

The events of the war, the conditions it imposed on the nation, and the various social forces of the prewar and war years—all were to lead to a severe nursing shortage that became acute immediately after the war and persisted at high levels until the late 1970s. Peak shortages, virtual crises, occurred in the late 1950s and early 1960s. The discussions of the shortage at the time and since have been numerous, and the economic and social issues the shortage entails are enormously complex. Our concern here, however, is not with the details of the shortage nor whether a given explanation of its causes and cure might be correct.

Instead, our concern is with the sheer fact of the shortage. The pressures it exerted on health and educational officials at the time affected nursing education dramatically. The ADN movement took form in the crucible of a persistent fear that the nation was not recruiting and educating enough young people to provide the nurses we would need.

A few experts believed that the return of nurses from military duty in 1945 would produce an excess of nurses seeking employment in civilian health care, but nursing shortages continued unabated after the war.[26] In 1946 the National Nursing Council (as it was by then known) projected the nation's need for nurses to be 359,500, the current supply to be 317,800, and so anticipated a shortage of 41,700.[27] This number assumed that 37,900 nurses released from military service after 1 September 1945 would be available for active service in civilian health care. Many military nurses, of course, did not in fact continue in active practice at war's end. Also in 1946 the USPHS, the Commonwealth Study Fund, and the AHA estimated nursing shortages, ranging from 75,000 too few nurses in the hospitals to 130,600 too few in the general health care delivery system.[28]

The nursing shortage, whatever its size may have been, is also reflected in the statistics about shutdowns in the nation's hospitals: in 1947, 32,000 hospital beds were closed, and in 1951, 14,000 were still not available to patients because of lack of nursing staff. In 1951 the nursing shortage was estimated to be 49,200, and by 1953 the number was raised to an unprecedented 65,000.[29]

Federal assistance to nursing students through the Cadet Nurse program had caused the number of annual graduations to increase dramatically. In 1940 the number of yearly graduations was 23,600, but by 1946 the number had increased by 12,595. Without federal aid the number of nursing graduates fell precipitously. In 1949 the number of graduates was smaller than in the last prewar year.[30]

Two concerns came up repeatedly: why weren't more students choosing nursing as a career, and why weren't more licensed nurses continuing in active service after the first few years following graduation? The postwar shortage prompted the federal government to examine these issues. The Department of Labor conducted an extensive survey of 21,000 nurses from all states, examining the characteristics of the profession, marking out regional variations, and looking at nurses' living conditions, benefits, and attitudes toward work; it compared its findings with similar facts about other fields.[31] In assessing the earnings and working conditions of such a large sample, the government laid bare a basic problem: nursing was facing stiff competition from other career fields then opening up for women. The war, among other things, profoundly affected the status of women in the labor market, and young women now had more options than before the war. The arduous life of both the student and the registered nurse had become a negative factor affecting the choices of many young women.[32]

The advances in medicine and surgery, as well as the emergence of specialization, were basic factors propelling the increasing demand for RNs. The increase was also fueled by the rapid growth in the number of hospitals and hospital beds, a result of the stimulus of the Hill-Burton Act.

By the end of the 1940s, then, conditions were ripe for the emergence of a wholly new, unprecedented way to educate registered nurses. Everywhere, there was the perception that nurses were scarce and that the shortage would not just go away. Americans were more than ever focused on education as a means of solving social problems and optimistic about their ability to succeed in applying such solutions. At the same time, they had become acutely aware of the new demand for nursing services in a rapidly expanding health care system. The nation needed to maintain the number and quality of nurses to sustain its growth.

Some of the short-term measures adopted during the war to meet defense emergencies provided models that might be followed. Americans had found that nursing education could be abbreviated and had experimented with the use of sundry nursing assistants. Ferment in the nursing profession itself signaled impending change; organizing more coherently now at the national level, nursing leaders saw new means to steer nursing in the directions that nurses themselves wanted. Primary among these goals was the movement of nursing education away from the control of individual hospitals and into the general system of American higher education.

Setting the Stage for a New

Nursing Program

At the end of the war, government officials, physicians, hospital administrators, educators, and nursing leaders were working on plans for reform that would improve American health care and the education of health care professionals. Many of these efforts would coalesce into the ADN movement, for it became increasingly apparent to many during the last half of the 1940s that by educating nurses in two-year colleges the nation might resolve the concerns of nurses and others about the future directions of nursing education and at the same time address the nurse shortage problem.

In June 1945 a meeting was held at the U.S. Office of Education in Washington to explore the expanded uses of the junior college, but no nurses were included and nursing education was not on the agenda—to the consternation of members of the board of the NLNE. One board member reported to her colleagues, moreover, that the American Association of Junior Colleges (AAJC) was then discussing the inclusion of nursing in junior college curricula. The NLNE, having no desire to be left out of further considerations of this possibility, authorized in January of 1946 the formation of a committee of its own to consider the development of nursing programs in junior colleges. The league's committee would include representatives of the Association of Collegiate Schools of Nursing (ACSN).[1]

Nursing leaders, of course, had for many years pushed to remove nursing education from the control of service agencies. Typically, their efforts had been opposed by physicians' and hospital administrators' groups, which argued that the nurses were exhibiting little more than self-interest. Now, however, with the pressure building everywhere for a solution to the nursing shortage, nursing had a better chance than ever before to bring about the educational reforms its leaders had envisioned for so long. The NLNE board was therefore interested in far more than developing just junior-college nursing education; the league's overall goal was to make nursing education collegiate wherever possible.

By 1947, a year before the Brown Report, it had developed a strong enough consensus to issue a position paper formally proposing that nursing education be moved out of the hospital and into the system of higher education and that the league support efforts to bring about the change. "Education of professional nurses should be an integral part of an institution of higher education, either public or private, or should be in a school conducted as an independent institution empowered by the state to grant appropriate degrees," asserted the league. It further declared that "the majority of schools in the country are controlled and administered by hospitals, which are service agencies. It is urged that such schools give early consideration to the transfer of control and administration to educational institutions." The paper argued that nursing students should have the opportunity to use educational facilities equal to those of students preparing for other fields of "social endeavor."[2] The paper expressed only the board's position at this time; it was not until the 1950 convention that the entire membership formally adopted this stand. In the meantime it faced the opposition of the AMA and the AHA.

Foundation Interest

Though they had opposition, nurses were not alone in proposing that nursing education become collegiate. A growing number of foundations were becoming concerned in the years following the war that nursing was not keeping pace with the demand for its services. In many instances it was the nursing shortages that triggered foundation officials' concern. They saw a strong connection between the quality of nursing services and the quality of nurses' education, and they typically sought solutions in educational reform.

The Commonwealth Fund, for example, funded the Commission on Hospital Care. The commission formed shortly after the war to draft guidelines for the tremendous postwar hospital expansion that was widely anticipated. The commission's twenty-two members included two nurses, an educator, and a hospital administrator. Its recommendations for nursing education included reducing the number of nursing schools, moving as many as possible into colleges and larger hospitals, and finding ways to reduce the time required to complete the general nursing course.[3]

The impact on nursing as a whole and the nursing education reform that would result from Kellogg's involvement with the National Nursing Council and, through it, with the national nursing organizations and other foundations would be very hard to measure, but it is safe to say that in the long run the impact grew to be considerable. Together, the people from the organizations, the foundations, and educational leaders serving on university faculties built the impetus behind the critically important Brown Report.

In praise of the National Nursing Council, Emory W. Morris, president and general director of the Kellogg Foundation, pointed out: "Significant strides in planning for nursing on the national level were made during the war and for the short period immediately following the war" thanks to the existence of the council. Kellogg believed that "groups within the nursing framework had to work together under strong leadership . . . to progress efficiently and at the same time quickly." To that end, the foundation had contributed $331,500 to the council during the war, in effect helping to promote closer cooperation among the six leading national nursing organizations: NLNE, ANA, NOPHN, NACGN, ACSN, and NAIN.[4]

The crisis in health care brought on by the war and the experience gained by the federal government in administering the funds for the Cadet Nurse Corps had exposed the basic, underlying weaknesses in nursing education to a wider public than ever before. The nursing leaders in the council, realizing that the widespread worry over the nursing shortage provided them with the opportunity to gain broader support for the educational changes long sought by nursing, recommended that a national study be made of nursing education, "with emphasis on the organization, administration, and control of schools of nursing."[5] Using funds provided for the task by the Carnegie Foundation, the council engaged a member of the staff of the Russell Sage Foundation, social anthropologist Dr. Esther Lucile Brown. Her assignment was to study nursing, just as she had studied other American occupations as a Sage researcher. Dr. Brown conducted her study during the fall, winter, and spring of 1947 and 1948, meeting with nursing leaders in conferences and visiting more than fifty schools.[6]

The published report of her study, formally titled *Nursing for the Future* but quickly dubbed the Brown Report, appeared in September

1948.[7] It became the rallying point for nurse reformers, who welcomed the corroboration of their views by a social scientist and by the foundations that had sponsored her work.

In her report Brown argued that the United States should be educating its nurses at least as well as it was educating its teachers at the nation's colleges and universities. She further criticized hospital-based programs as inadequate and authoritarian, and she argued that such programs would have increasing difficulty attracting newcomers to the nursing field. She pointed out that acute shortages, old-fashioned educational methods, low salaries for nurses, and the low esteem in which nurses and nurse educators were held were drastically reducing the number of women who were choosing nursing as a career. Brown recommended the establishment of nursing schools to match the number of the nation's medical schools and to be distributed throughout the country in colleges and universities. A sound system of accreditation for those schools was also needed, she insisted.[8]

Once the report was published, the National Nursing Council as such reached the end of its formal existence. But the representatives of the member organizations saw to it that organized nursing would continue to cooperate at the national level to push for reform. The council was replaced by a group known as the Committee to Implement the Brown Report, which consisted of representatives from the same six national nursing organizations that had formed the core of the original council, as well as other interested parties. The organizations contributed funds, and a chairman, a member of the faculty at Teachers College, Columbia University, was appointed. The profession was organizing for a major push toward nursing educational reform.

Soon after its formation, the Committee to Implement the Brown Report approached the W. K. Kellogg Foundation to ask for funds to convene a group of leading citizens to help the committee formulate a national program for improving nursing education. The request was turned down. After arranging for consultation between committee leaders and an expert in higher education from Teachers College, Kellogg officers concluded that the nursing leaders were still too isolated from the leaders in other fields, too immersed in the daily pressures of their immediate jobs, to be able to present their cause to the nation's policymakers. Kellogg, however, recognized the urgent need to implement the recommendations of the Brown Report, and so it decided instead to provide the means for nursing leaders and their national organizations to receive the help they needed to carry out their mission.[9]

Its first step was to sponsor a five-day conference held 4–11 January 1949 in Battle Creek to discuss the issues raised in the Brown Report and to formulate a beginning plan that the nursing organizations could carry out. Among the consultants made available to the implementation committee members were a handful of nursing leaders, the members of the foundation's Education Advisory Committee and its Nursing Advisory Committee (in other words, the consultants in these fields that the foundation relied on), and key people in higher education, including four persons from Teachers College, Columbia University. Dr. Hollis Caswell of Columbia had suggested to the foundation prior to the meeting that leaders in higher education generally should be mobilized to help nursing develop its plan.[10]

The conference identified the key issues of the Brown Report under these headings: collegiate schools of nursing; hospital schools of nursing; technical schools of nursing; legislation, accreditation, and financing; and total planning.[11] Its division of nursing schools into three groups, with "technical" specified as the third type, is a clear indication of the drift that events were taking.

The conference in January sparked activity in many quarters. For example, Dr. Donald Young, general director of the Russell Sage Foundation, called a meeting of sixteen officials of major American foundations to review the Brown Report and the Battle Creek conference to discover what types of projects in nursing education the private agencies might pursue. That meeting was held at Carnegie Foundation headquarters on 24 February 1949. Among the foundations represented besides Carnegie, Russell Sage, and Kellogg were the Buhl Foundation, the Commonwealth Fund, the Ford Foundation, the Knapp Foundation, the Josiah Macy Foundation, the John and Mary R. Markle Foundation, the A. W. Mellon Educational and Charitable Trust, the Milbank Memorial Fund, the Elisabeth Severance Prentiss Foundation, the Rockefeller Foundation, and the Helen Hay Whitney Foundation. It became clear during the meeting that of all the foundations, the Rockefeller and Kellogg programs had the most highly developed interests in nursing service and education. The consensus of the officials was that nursing was at the same kind of turning point that medicine had experienced in 1910, when the Flexner Report was completed and major reforms in medical education in the United States were begun. "The next five to ten years," averred the Kellogg director's report back to Kellogg, "will provide a real opportunity for constructive work in this field."[12]

The meeting stimulated action by several of the foundations. The Russell Sage Foundation announced that it would place a full-time person on its staff to advise institutions of higher education about the types of nursing programs that would be needed. The Kellogg Foundation's Nursing Division began planning its future efforts in helping to improve nursing service and education. Immediately following the war the foundation had designated $979,436 for a program assisting ten universities to establish or expand existing nursing programs to meet the needs of nurses newly separated from the service or whose civilian jobs during the war had prevented or interrupted their advanced educational plans. On 29 and 30 November 1949 the foundation invited the project directors to meet with the foundation's advisory group in nursing to review the forty projects at the ten sites and to discuss future directions their efforts might take.[13]

In the meantime, the reorganized Committee to Implement the Brown Report, now named the Committee for the Improvement of Nursing Services, was moving forward with its plans. Members of the committee had returned to their respective organizations to explain the committee's long-range goals and to organize support from within the profession. The committee asked for and in September received $7,000 from the Rockefeller Foundation to maintain a small staff until July 1950. Marian Sheahan, formerly the director of public health nursing for the New York State Health Department, was employed as the committee's director. Kellogg officials expected that a reinvigorated and better organized committee would be able to formulate an overall plan of nursing education reform that the foundation could support.[14]

Through the winter and into summer of 1950, the foundation and nursing leaders worked to refine their plans. Ultimately, the Kellogg people were impressed enough with the progress being made by the committee and by the proposals it brought forward to approve a commitment of up to $200,000 over a three-year period to help "activate" its program.[15] Payments were to be made to the NLNE, which had agreed to act as the administrative agency for the implementation committee; the funds were designated for the use of the committee to meet its basic operational expenses for a headquarters staff.[16]

The committee established three important subcommittees: on education, on nursing service, and on accreditation. Twenty-eight states formed their own Committees for the Improvement of Nursing Services, and regional-level action was yet another goal.

Accreditation and Educational Reform

The work begun on accreditation under the aegis of this group was one of its more important contributions to nursing education reform. With the institution of nationally recognized accreditation standards and procedures, nursing could hope to see an end to poor, weak programs, wherever they might be based, and the more vigorous development of better programs, whether cast in traditional molds or developed along more innovative lines.

For its efforts in developing a system of accreditation, the committee received support from many sources other than the Kellogg Foundation: the Commonwealth Fund contributed $75,000; the National Foundation for Infantile Paralysis, $61,250; and the Rockefeller Foundation, $65,000. Another $100,000 was expected from nurses themselves, through income received for registration fees they would pay to attend regional conferences on accreditation.[17] By 1951 progress had been made toward the goal of instituting a national system for accrediting nursing education programs. The National Nursing Accrediting Service initiated its School Improvement Program that year, appointing Helen Nahm to head the project. Plans called for self-study by individual schools, consultation to schools seeking to become accredited, and the identification of common problems.[18]

A critical part of the accreditation drive was the School Data Analysis Project, the purpose of which was to provide the information needed to establish a "unified accrediting service" for all nursing schools.[19] The Brown Report had strongly recommended the institution of national accrediting for nursing schools, and there was wide agreement among health care delivery experts that some such means of controlling the quality of nursing schools was much needed. The system for educating nurses still in place at the end of the 1940s was archaic, for it had little to do with modern teaching theory and practice. Owned and operated by the hospital, the nursing school offered apprenticeship training; and although apprenticeships in the health care occupations had made sense in an earlier America, such an approach was hardly appropriate in the context of modern scientific health care practice. During World War II the nursing students in the nation's hospitals were providing the lion's share, 60 to 80 percent, of patient care by nurses; in the postwar years as the nursing shortage grew more acute, the student nurses continued to provide a large share of many a community's hospital manpower. The situation was exploitive, in the opinion of nursing leaders.

In November 1949 a preliminary report of the nursing school survey was published by the ANA in the *American Journal of Nursing*.[20] Lucile Petry and her coauthors described the design of ten state surveys and several community studies intended to measure existing nursing resources, estimate future needs of health programs, and suggest a plan for nursing education to meet those needs. The findings confirmed the extent of the nursing shortage. The authors argued that the expansion of nursing education needed to be very carefully planned, especially on the regional level, and that nursing had to overcome what they called the "emotional blocks" to reorganization in nursing education.

The full report of the survey was published in 1950 under the title *Nursing Schools at the Mid-Century*. It corroborated the findings of the Brown Report and the arguments of the reformist literature that had begun to appear in response to the report.[21] Of the 1,193 schools surveyed by the project, 97 percent had responded. What the researchers found was alarming: only 25 percent of the schools met the standards set in 1939 for nursing schools; 50 percent did less well than that, more nearly meeting standards set ten years earlier in 1929; and the remaining 25 percent ranked lower still. The report found that collegiate programs generally were the superior schools and voiced a formal call for the accreditation of all nursing schools. The authors projected that "it would probably cost an additional ten to fifteen million a year to raise the standards of instruction in all schools to the average level of those in . . . the top 25 percent."[22]

In 1949 a total of 88,817 students were enrolled in nursing schools: 82,182 of these young people were attending hospital schools of nursing
and only 6,635 were in "collegiate" programs.[23] Montag warns that not even these many nursing students were actually attending college, however, for the term "collegiate" was carefully chosen to cover much more than degree-granting programs. Many of the so-called collegiate programs did not lead to the baccalaureate; they represented only the numerous ad hoc arrangements by which a student in a hospital program might take a course or two at a local college. A nursing school's connection to a college could be quite tenuous, and the nursing programs often bore little resemblance to other undergraduate programs at the college.[24]

Two full-length reports were now circulating nationally and stirring up a virtual fever of reform. The Brown Report and *Nursing Schools at the Mid-Century*, in their portrayals of nurses themselves and of their schools, not only corroborated one another, they galvanized nurses and their allies in education into action. And the nursing shortage, now looming into crisis proportions, continued to prompt many others to lend their support.

Developing Professional Standards for Practice

The Committee for the Improvement of Nursing Services director Marian Sheahan invited a representative group of leaders to New York to meet 1–3 March 1950 to discuss nursing's most pressing needs and to obtain suggestions for use in drafting the formal plans of the Committee for the Improvement of Nursing Services. (Funds for this final push toward an action proposal were provided by Kellogg, which would also underwrite the program that the proposal outlined.) Besides the six nursing organizations sponsoring the committee, representatives of the AMA, the AHA, the Catholic Hospital Association, and the American Council of Education attended the meeting.

The group worked out details for a plan of action: field studies were to be conducted at both the state and the regional levels to (1) determine the number of nurses that were needed, (2) assess the adequacy of current nursing practice, and (3) project the kinds of nursing needed, as determined by the conditions seen among hospital patients. A national clearinghouse for these studies would be established. Moreover, hospitals were to be encouraged to conduct self-studies and to make the periodic evaluation of nursing services an integral part of in-service education for staff. The result, it was hoped, would be to define nursing functions, to eliminate non-nursing work from the staff nurse's duties, and to have nursing service directors closely monitoring nursing duties and functions. Finally, the committee strongly backed the notion of advanced education for nursing administrators and supervisors. Committee members expected that state and local workshops based on the program they outlined would garner widespread support for their plans.[25]

The strategy of the committee was expressed by its name: the hope was that by focusing first on the improvement of nursing service, they could make a stronger case for the improvement of education for nurses. Their plan was designed to counter the criticism that nursing leaders had confronted so often in the past, that their pressure for the reform of nursing education was self-seeking careerism that would little benefit patients. The committee hoped that a detailed analysis of actual nursing practice would show the public that the need for educational reform was indeed acute.

In the end, the committee hoped, they would have sampled good nursing practice, defined it, and then developed standards of practice that could be followed by all. The standards would be field-tested at selected hospitals, and guidelines would be developed, which could be further refined for evaluating nursing practice. The committee could thus supply the evaluation forms and consultative services to individual hospitals requesting the service. This plan, like the plan for national nursing school accreditation, expressed a need that was strongly felt among nursing leaders at this juncture. Until universal standards for both nursing education and nursing practice could be established, "professional" nursing would be more a hope than a reality. Until an occupation can be defined by such universally recognized standards, it has little claim to the status of a profession.

Innovative Views of Nursing and Educational Reform

During 1947 Eli Ginzberg of Columbia University directed the work of a university group concerned with the nursing crisis, the Committee on the Functions of Nursing, which met in six sessions at Teachers College, Columbia, to discuss materials that Ginzberg distributed in advance of each meeting. The group identified several factors that contributed to the nursing shortage. It saw the shortage as "jeopardizing the entire structure of medical care" and affecting every facet of nursing service,[26] and it predicted that critical nursing shortages could not be overcome without the institution of two tiers of practitioners in nursing, one of them professional, the other technical. Ginzberg's committee based its recommendation on the notion that nursing functions extend along a continuum from the simplest to the most complex, a conception that suggests the designation of portions of the range to different groups of workers. The committee's overall conception was undoubtedly the basis for Mildred Montag's doctoral research a year or two later, conducted under the direction of the Teachers College faculty. The work of Ginzberg's committee is evidence of a crucial development: nursing and educational leaders were beginning to ana-

lyze the work of the nurse so as to find ways to break out of the traditional mold and develop new structures that would fit modern practice
in hospitals and other agencies giving care. Nursing might be viewed as
a whole set of roles and functions, not just the single one defined earlier.

That innovative ideas such as these of the Ginzberg committee
should be emanating from Teachers College at this time was no accident. The college by the 1940s had established a reputation as a pioneer
in nursing education. The school was, for example, attracting the support of the Kellogg Foundation, whose officials chose to underwrite a
key program of Teachers College in the belief that an investment in this
school would have "wide implications" because it was "an international
center in nursing education."[27] From 1945 to 1949 Kellogg provided
nearly $80,000 to finance the expansion of the Teachers College gradu-
ate program, which focused on educating nurses who would become
faculty members and administrators of basic collegiate nursing programs.
The ambitious project included a comprehensive study of the overall
nursing curriculum by the college faculty. Directing the project for the
college was a faculty member who would figure prominently in the
ADN movement: Dr. R. Louise McManus.[28]

Columbia University was not alone in promoting the AD idea. In
1950 the NLNE board approached the AAJC, suggesting that a committee be formed by the league, the AAJC, and the ACSN to study nursing
education. In effect, the league was asking the national leaders in junior
college education to formally study and consider the recommendations
of the Brown Report. At the time, some eighty or so arrangements
between junior colleges and hospital schools of nursing were in existence, plans by which the colleges supplied instruction in the social
and biological sciences and in certain humanities courses. In short, the
junior colleges were not wholly without experience in nursing education, though no freestanding junior-college nursing programs were in
existence.

By May of 1950 the NLNE representatives on the joint committee
were ready to report their findings to the NLNE board about the potential for nursing education in junior and community colleges. One program suggestion emerging from these earliest meetings was for a two-
year program in nursing with transfer at the end of two years to a senior
university. Another was for a three-year program that would culminate
in an associate of arts or science degree and that would qualify the
graduate for RN licensure.[29]

The NLNE board responded by asking the group to meet again. Funds designated for the National Committee for the Improvement of Nursing Services were to cover the cost of adding members to the AAJC-NLNE joint committee.

In the months that followed, the joint committee developed plans for several activities. First, they would survey junior colleges to determine their interest in establishing nursing programs. From among those expressing interest, the committee would select five to serve as pilot projects in this new kind of nursing education. Nursing leaders would be used as consultants to guide the development of the new programs and to evaluate the results. At this time, in 1950, the committee was particularly interested in three roles in nursing education for the junior college: educating practical nurses, providing an associate degree in nursing that could serve ultimately as the base for a baccalaureate degree in nursing, and providing in-service training for hospital nursing staffs.[30]

The NLNE board quickly approved a national advisory committee on experimental nursing programs in junior colleges. Representatives from the league, ACSN, and AAJC were charged with preparing guidelines for program development, obtaining the funds to pay for consulting services, and securing financing for the pilot program itself.[31]

The year 1950 was a landmark year for the associate degree in nursing. As work among nursing leaders in the national organizations and educational leaders in their associations moved ever closer to the ADN idea, Mildred Montag, a doctoral student at Columbia University, was completing the research for and writing her dissertation. Here at Teachers College, under the direction of faculty that had put forth some of the most creative thinking of the postwar period about the nurse's function and education, she worked out the philosophy and plan for an entirely new kind of nursing program, developing at the same time the design for research that would test the viability of the idea.

The proposal broke with the seventy-five-year-old stereotyped pattern of preparation for nursing which was work-centered and hospital-centered. It took into account the changing needs of society for nursing service, the changing emphasis in medical care. It proposed a technical worker in nursing, more limited *in scope* than professional nursing but broader in scope than that of practical nursing. It should be noted that up to that time practical nurse schools had not played a significant role in the scheme of nursing education. The proposal also took into account the development of community colleges and the need for nursing education to be within the established educational framework.[32]

The notion that had surfaced first in the Ginzberg committee's recommendations—that nursing functions might be divisible into levels—and that now found a variant expression in the educational plan outlined in Montag's work, was making itself felt in other places as well. The next year, 1951, would see the appointment of Mildred Montag to the NLNE-AAJC joint committee.

The efforts of nursing leaders to engage the support of professional educators were beginning to bear fruit. In April 1951 the Sixth Annual Conference of the National Education Association unanimously adopted a resolution that colleges and universities recognize a responsibility for establishing programs of professional and technical education of nurses. Clearly, not only was the idea that basic nursing education be made collegiate gaining wider acceptance, but so, too, was the idea that such nursing education might have a separate "technical" aspect.

Slowly but surely, all the pieces were being put in place. Professional nursing and higher education were in a state of full readiness for the first attempts to educate RNs in two-year programs based in junior and community colleges.

The Cooperative Research Project:

The ADN Pioneers

Mildred Montag's dissertation, *Education for Nursing Technicians,* might have languished on library shelves, as so many research reports do, were it not for the fact that this doctoral researcher had conducted her work under the direction of a faculty intent on finding better ways to educate more nurses. Montag's ideas about a two-year program became the center of an ambitious plan to mount and then test a model for an entirely new nursing degree. In large part because of the foresight and support of faculty members such as R. Louise McManus, director of the program at Teachers College, Columbia University, Montag's plan was translated into reality. It was McManus, for example, who brought the idea to those who provided the funds that made the initial pilot program possible.

Dr. McManus described the factors that came together to make the ADN program a reality:

> Seldom has there been a more fortuitous juxtaposition of (1) "an idea whose time has come" and a well-thought out philosophy, plan and proposal for research and experimentation; (2) the availability of a competent researcher, eager to undertake the project; (3) the offer of financial support from an anonymous donor who was eager to help assure better nursing services for America through improving education for nurses; and (4) a milieu in which the policies of the college permitted its resources and the experience of its faculty to be brought to bear upon the full accomplishment of the purpose of the research.[1]

January 1952 saw the formal beginning of the Cooperative Research Project (CRP) in Junior and Community College Education for Nursing, based at Teachers College, Columbia University. The identity of the "anonymous donor" McManus so discreetly described remains a secret carefully guarded by Dr. Montag. The $110,000 that launched the project was the gift of a group of women, not of an institution or foundation.[2] The project was to be directed by Dr. Montag, the "eager" researcher referred to by Dr. McManus. The project design reflected her doctoral research, but the project and the philosophy animating it were deeply rooted in the deliberations and events described in the preceding chapter.

Exploration of the Underlying Assumptions of the Project

The project had two controlling purposes: to define a new worker in nursing, the "technical" nurse, and then to design the educational preparation of this new kind of nurse. This nurse would be distinguished from other nurses by the scope of her practice. Her functions would fall somewhere between those of the practical nurse and those of the traditional professional nurse who was being educated in baccalaureate programs.

The project was based on four assumptions. The first, and most significant, was that the practice of nursing was not static; on the contrary, it was constantly changing and it was also becoming more complex. If nursing could be viewed as existing along a continuum or as having a spectrum of functions, then nursing functions could be viewed as ranging from the simple at one end of the continuum to the complex at the other end. That is, nursing aides might be described as functioning at one end and the nurse clinicians at the other. Between these two extremes, the most simple and the most advanced, exists an intermediate, or technical, array of knowledges and abilities that could be subsumed under a role to be defined and assigned to a new kind of nurse. Moreover, the CRP staff assumed that "the major number of nursing functions lay in the intermediate range."[3]

The closely following assumption was that an educational program could be developed to prepare this new nurse at the intermediate level. The precise functions assigned to the new role would define the content of the educational program.

The project also assumed that the nurse functioning at the simplest, most basic level could be prepared on the job and would not be a concern of the project research. Finally, it was assumed that the educational program should be conducted in an educational institution whose mission included the preparation of other technical workers—namely, a junior or community college.[4]

The selection of the junior college was paramount to the success of the project, but it was not a surprising choice. To understand why, one needs to know something of the history of the junior college idea in American education.

Today we think of the community college as a distinctively late-twentieth-century development, but in fact its origins are older than that. The basic American attitude toward education, the desire for extended universal education regardless of social position, family income, religious choice, or ethnic or racial background, would propel some public school systems solidly into the junior college movement as early as the 1920s.

The cornerstone of public higher education in America is the Morrill Act. Passed in 1862, the act awarded the states federally owned land that, when sold, would provide funds for each state to establish colleges devoted to the agricultural and mechanical arts. The Morrill Act set policies and practices for federal support for higher education that still prevail. Two purposes are fundamental: providing low-cost college education for many persons and offering a nonsectarian, nonclassical curriculum. With the establishment of the land-grant colleges during the years following the Civil War, the nation's public schools for the first time provided advanced instruction in the practical vocations and the applied sciences necessary to improve the quality of life of American citizens.

Ideological ferment in American university circles near the turn of the century found expression in a number of developments, the most important of which (for our story) is that most unique of American institutions, the junior college. Two Californians—Alexis F. Lange, dean of the School of Education of the University of California from 1906 to 1924, and David Starr Jordan, president of Leland Stanford University —were particularly influential in that movement. Like their colleagues at other universities, these two men were desirous of reserving for the university the best of the German and British traditions in scholarship and research. To accomplish this, they thought it best to channel the beginning and less able students into other institutions than the university. Other university leaders besides Lange and Jordan believed that a university education to prepare persons for careers as scholars should be separated from the rest of higher education. Among those influenced by the German university system were the presidents of a number of midwestern state universities, most notably William Rainey Harper of the University of Chicago. But it was the Californians who moved first to take steps to give their ideas concrete form on a statewide basis.

Lange and Jordan sought state legislation to permit California high schools to assume educational responsibility for the beginning college students. As early as 1892 the University of California had advocated the placement of the first two university years in secondary schools and smaller colleges; it also had accepted for full credit high school postsecondary courses.[5] Then, through Lange's and Jordan's efforts and the collaboration of public school officials, California in the early 1900s became the first state to pass legislation authorizing the establishment of local community colleges. In addition, a law passed in 1907 permitting high school boards of education to provide the first two university years by offering postsecondary courses in high school. In 1910 Fresno established the first public junior college in the state, under the leadership of Superintendent C. L. McLane.[6]

Encouraged by the headway they were making, Jordan by 1912 was looking forward to the time when the large high schools and small colleges of the state would relieve the large universities from the necessity of giving instruction of the first two university years. Superintendent McLane pledged in May of 1912 his support of both the University of California and Stanford University in their development of junior colleges.[7]

Lange continued to speak out on behalf of the new structure. Speaking at a university conference on secondary schools in 1917, he declared that the "state university, embodying in a higher indissoluble union the German and English university aims, rests on the foundation of fourteen grades of elementary and secondary education, its first two years corresponding to the last two years of the four-year college." No doubt reflecting the recent legislation in California, he continued: the university "retains the last two years of secondary education for a gradually diminishing number of students."[8]

But Lange went much further than most American advocates of the German model when in the same talk he described the purposes of the new junior college as promoting the general welfare, "which is the sole reason for its existence." Such colleges cannot make preparation for the university the "excuse for being," he asserted. Their curricula should be terminal rather than college preparatory. In this last declaration, he voiced an idea well ahead of its time.

Despite California's commitment to the junior college and the strong support for the idea in other scattered locations, the movement toward the German model was not fully realized in the United States at this time. Social factors combined to defeat the idea. The tradition that attached the first two postsecondary years to the university remained strong, and the American university retained essentially the same structure it had always had, except that its first two years were increasingly organized as a junior division.

Harper of Chicago had suggested three ways that the junior colleges could be created, but only one was destined to have any success in this country: the extension of the high school to include the first two years of collegiate work. Harper did separate freshmen and sophomores at the University of Chicago to create a lower division called a "junior college" in 1896. But then he set up a system of affiliated colleges in connection with an academy or secondary school, also calling these "junior colleges."[9] But, according to one writer, the "community college literature provides scant information on how local community colleges" like those in Chicago started.[10] Most developed as a result of the efforts of parents and sympathetic community leaders and school board members who desired greater opportunities for high school graduates in their communities. But little information about these pilot programs was issued publicly, apparently for fear of a backlash from taxpayers.

Nevertheless, it was just such extension of the public secondary schools that became the basis for the establishment of tax-supported junior colleges. Egalitarian goals, not elitism, were the motive that spelled eventual success for the junior college movement. What won the day was the practice of local control and support of free educational systems, extended to cover the first two college years for the sake of the less affluent and less scholarly students.[11]

For many years, only in California was the junior-college movement highly visible. In 1921 the California legislature authorized the establishment of junior college districts. These were to be established if a minimum high school population of 400 and a minimum assessed valuation of $10 million was present. California thereby moved into the forefront of the movement rapidly during the 1920s. By 1930, according to Fields, "California had enrolled fifteen thousand students in thirty-four junior colleges, or about half of the total community college enrollment throughout the nation and about half of the total college enrollment in California institutions of higher education."[12]

Another major development in the junior college movement came after the end of World War II. The war itself seemed to have released a tide of rising expectations among Americans whose social, racial, and ethnic backgrounds had long permitted them to foster only modest hopes. Now, braced by educational benefits from the federal government, former servicemen and -women flocked home—and to school. The Truman administration responded quickly to the consequent pressure for more education for more people. Truman appointed the President's Commission on Higher Education and placed at its head George F. Zook, a longtime friend of the junior college and president of the American Council on Education. According to one historian of the movement, the report of this commission is "one of the more famous federal documents on American education."[13]

After establishing that at least 49 percent of the population had the mental ability to complete fourteen years of schooling in curricula leading to employment or further study, the commission said:

> To be sure of its own health and strength a democratic society must provide free and equal access to education for its youth, and at the same time it must recognize their differences in capacity and purpose. Higher education in America should include a variety of institutional forms and educational programs, so that at whatever point any student leaves school, he will be fitted, within the limits of his mental capacity and educational level, for an abundant and productive life as a person, a worker, and as a citizen.
>
> As one means of achieving the expansion of educational opportunity and the diversification of educational offerings it considers necessary, this Commission recommends that the number of community colleges be increased and that their activities be multiplied.[14]

The commission's use of the name "community" college was no accident. Because Zook and many members of the commission were advocates of schools that would strengthen democracy and increase opportunity, they believed that the "junior" college should break away from its fascination with preparing students for transfer to senior colleges and instead devote more energy and resources to the development of two-year terminal programs. Here, after many years, Lange's pioneering idea of 1917 found official expression, at the national level. The commission explained its position:

preparatory programs looking to the more advanced courses of the senior college are not complete and rounded in themselves, and they usually do not serve well the purpose of those who must terminate their schooling at the end of the fourteenth grade. Half the young people who go to college find themselves unable to complete the full 4-year course, and for a long time to come more students will end their formal education in the junior college years than will prolong it into the senior college. These 2-year graduates would gain more from a terminal program planned specifically to meet their needs than from the first half of a 4-year curriculum. For this reason, the Commission recommends that the community college emphasize programs of terminal education.[15]

The commission advocated the publicly and locally controlled multi-purpose, two-year college as *the* model for the new community college. Though locally oriented, the community colleges should be "carefully planned to fit into a comprehensive Statewide system of higher education," declared the commissioners.[16] Their financial support would come primarily from the local community but would be supplemented by state funds.

The commission envisioned much for the community college. Foreseeing continual change, it argued that the community college would need to be ever ready to adapt its programs to meet current needs. Foreseeing a growing tendency among older students to alternate periods of attendance and remunerative work, it promoted the idea that these colleges offer cooperative education programs attuned to the needs of business and industry. Foreseeing the possibility of the development of a two-tiered program consisting of liberal and vocational educations that would produce "workers" and "citizens," the commission warned that the community college must make the effort to maintain a well-integrated single program. Finally, anticipating increasing specialization in many fields, the commission warned that the college, to remain viable, would have to meet the needs of students who would go on to more specialized or professional study even as it focused on its terminal programs.[17] All of these points would have great importance later for the ADN program, as subsequent events would prove.

Central to the commission's work was its strongly democratic focus. It saw the community college as the best way for American higher education to expand its programs and services to meet the needs of a widening array of citizens. It saw "service to the entire community" as the central purpose of the community college, which would "remove geographic and economic barriers to educational opportunity and discover and develop individual talents at low cost and easy access."[18] Such a purpose fit the times; these were the immediate postwar years, when the nation's economy was on the upswing and the renewed focus on domestic needs was sparked by optimism.

Truman himself remained committed to the community college idea, as revealed in a letter he wrote to Oscar R. Ewing, administrator of the Federal Security Agency, in early 1950. He told Ewing that he planned to recommend in his budget message for 1950 a "limited Federal program to assist capable youth" who might otherwise not continue their higher educations. Moreover, he was "particularly interested in knowing more about the efforts to reduce geographic and economic barriers to the development of individual talents" by the community colleges. He asked that a comprehensive study of these colleges be conducted over the next six months; he wished particularly to have recommendations about whether the federal government should assist in the development of community colleges, and if so, what the best means for providing such assistance might be.[19]

Thus, the assumptions of those planning the Cooperative Research Project in Junior and Community College Education for Nursing, who were intent on demonstrating the worth of the ADN idea, were rooted in fertile soil. Given the widening interest in associate degree education, project planners could expect the two-year program to be met with support from a number of important directions, not the least of which was the federal government.

None of the project's four basic assumptions, taken alone, was new. Each had received considerable attention throughout the 1940s as concern grew over the ability of the health care system to stay abreast of scientific advance and the expanding health needs of the nation. What *was* new was the precise combination of the ideas into a plan of action.

That plan was unlike anything else in the history of nursing education. The CRP would not only design a new educational program for a new kind of worker, it would mount two-year pilot programs to prepare young people to perform those "intermediate" functions commonly assigned to the RN. The graduates of these new programs would qualify for licensure as RNs, meet the requirements of the junior college for a degree, be employable upon graduation, and be prepared to become fully competent practitioners (the expectation was that they would not be fully competent at graduation).

The Structure and Administration of the Project

An Advisory Committee for the project was formed, composed of nurse educators, community college educators, nursing and hospital administrators, and interested citizens. The group met annually to review the project's progress and to discuss with project staff ways to improve methods of operation. To stay informed, the committee visited project sites and talked with faculty members. One of the more important functions of the members of the committee was to keep their own separate constituencies fully informed about the project.

The project was centered in New York City, where the CRP staff was based. Dr. Mildred Montag was the director of the project. She was assisted by an educator whose expertise lay in community college development and administration: this position was held initially by Dr. Walter Sindlinger, a former dean of Orange County Community College in California, and later by two others, Dr. J. F. Marvin Buechel, former president of Everett Junior College in Washington, and Dr. Lassar G. Gotkin, an expert in evaluation who served during the final year of the project. The staff was expanded during the final year to include Alice R. Rines.

The plan called for the location of pilot programs in existing community colleges that expressed an interest in instituting the new program. By situating the experimental programs in schools that demonstrated an existing commitment to the ADN idea, the CRP could expect to devote its funds entirely to actual program start-up and could hope to see its pilot programs continue after the five-year project came to an end. By using community colleges located in different regions of the country (the project adopted districts as defined by the AAJC), CRP staff believed that the project could better test the efficacy of the program.

Colleges interested in participating in the project completed questionnaires eliciting basic information about the schools. Project leaders followed up with site visits to probable locations. As this work moved forward, the advisory committee refined the criteria for selecting the sites. To be included, a college had to demonstrate: (1) interest in a nursing program that would be a distinct departure from the traditional nursing program; (2) its community's need and readiness for such a program; (3) the assurance that control of the nursing program would rest with the college; (4) its financial ability to operate the program; (5) its faculty's acceptance of the idea; (6) the availability of the necessary learning resources, including clinical facilities in nearby hospitals, clinics, and agencies; (7) the existence of reasonable assurance that graduates could achieve licensure and find employment.[20]

The colleges that were ultimately selected to participate in the CRP and the years they joined the project are listed below:

Orange County Community College	1952
Middletown, New York	
Fairleigh Dickinson University	1952
Rutherford, New Jersey	
Henry Ford Community College	1953
Dearborn, Michigan	
Weber College	1953
Ogden, Utah	
Pasadena City College	1953
Pasadena, California	
Virginia Intermont College	1954
Bristol, Virginia	
Virginia State College, Norfolk Division	1955
Norfolk, Virginia	

Each of these schools represented a different organizational pattern, source of financial support, and student body composition. Virginia Intermont College, for example, was located on a residential campus and admitted only women. Pasadena City College, in contrast, was non-residential and coeducational. The program at each site was controlled and financed by the college, not by the project. Also, each college was responsible for selecting, approving, and paying its own faculty.

Developing the New Curriculum

The nursing faculty at each site was expected to develop a curriculum for its program that would complement the other programs at the college. Each faculty, as it worked on curriculum development, had the benefit of advice from the CRP staff, in addition to the stimulus and information provided at the summer workshops.

Dr. Montag had presented a model curriculum in her dissertation that was further modified by the CRP. The curriculum contained both general education and nursing courses. At the beginning of the project the mix was one-third general education and two-thirds nursing, but that ratio was later changed so that the balance was roughly half and half. The general education courses were the same as those taken by students in other college programs to meet the requirements for the associate degree.

At its first meeting, 12–23 March 1952, the advisory committee agreed on the following statement regarding the appropriate philosophy to animate the development of the new curriculum:

> [The] nursing curriculum will be developed around the knowledge of man, his development and behavior, contemporary society and its problems, including major health problems, and the specialized services which nursing should render in relation to human and social needs.[21]

The nursing courses at project sites thus were organized on a conception of nursing that was patient-centered, not disease-centered. This move away from the disease as the central focus was the element in the curriculum design that most clearly distinguished the new programs from traditional nursing education. The traditional programs based in the hospitals had been structured to follow clinical rotations through the specialties of medical practice (medicine, surgery, and so forth). The pilot programs in the CRP were organized on the basis of a "broad fields" conception of nursing content that reflected the everyday experiences of the staff nurse. Typical topics for courses were adult nursing, maternal and child health nursing, psychosocial nursing, or family nursing.

So important was the new approach to the project that the staff planned to devote the first summer workshop to the development of a "broad fields" curriculum plan for sites to use. Three basic curricular areas were identified at this meeting: the fundamentals of nursing, maternal and child care, and physical and mental illness. Faculty members who attended the workshop then returned to their respective sites to develop the individual courses based on these broad fields.

The first nursing course in any program on the fundamentals of nursing focused on "the needs of all persons based on the fundamental needs of man and the health guidance and nursing care appropriate to those needs." It was more than the usual introductory course, for the fundamentals covered here were repeated in later courses, when they were built upon and developed further. The second nursing course, also taught in the first year, was on maternal and child health. Its focus was the normal maternity cycle and the normal child.

The second year addressed deviations from the normal in the human life cycle, with an emphasis on illness and disease. The different faculties chose a variety of ways to organize this material. Usually, major health problems were the organizing principle, but each faculty was free to select its own method of presenting the material.

The basic program was designed to last two years, but a few of the project sites required four semesters whereas others required four semesters plus a summer session. Courses in the second year usually were "double in credits" to those of the first year. Summer sessions were typically an extension of the coursework in physical and mental illness.

The staff members visited each project site annually, to collect data to be used in the follow-up of graduates and to solicit ideas for the annual summer workshops for site participants. The subjects of the workshops included the development of the broad fields curriculum, the refinement of program objectives, the exploration of new learning opportunities for nursing students, teaching methods, and the evaluation of student performance.

Clinical Instruction in the New Program

Another marked departure of the new programs was their being much less centered in the hospital than the traditional nursing programs had been. The new programs used a variety of health care facilities to provide clinical instruction for their students. Hospitals remained the primary sources of clinical experience, but the students—now learners rather than laborers—attended other community facilities. The new sites chosen by faculties included day nurseries, nursing homes, specialized hospitals, health clinics, family planning agencies, public schools, physicians' offices, and self-help groups. Each facility was chosen with specific learning goals in mind.

Each project site developed a campus laboratory for the nursing program. Students could practice here their psychomotor skills and learn various processes and procedures at the college prior to or along with their experience at the hospital.

The combination of the college-based laboratory with the use of a variety of health facilities meant that a nursing faculty could plan and direct students' clinical learning with much more precision than had ever been possible in the hospital-based nursing programs. Theoretically, this meant that students could learn in a shorter time, for what was eliminated was both the needless repetition and the menial tasks that confronted the student nurse working nights and weekends on hospital wards. The former contributed little if anything to her learning, and the latter probably disrupted it.

The Students in the First Programs

The students who attended these pilot programs at the project sites were recruited and selected according to each college's admissions criteria; specialized criteria rather than open admissions policies were developed later, as the number of programs grew rapidly. These students contrasted markedly with the usual students in traditional nursing programs. To begin with, they were older. Their ages ranged from sixteen to fifty-nine, and 14 percent were over twenty-six years old. Hospital programs did not accept older students. Another difference was that more of the students in the new program were men; at a time when fewer than 1 percent of the admissions to hospital schools of nursing were male,[22] the new nursing programs were admitting three men for every one hundred students. Yet another difference: at a time when the traditional hospital-based nursing schools were prohibiting marriage for their students until the final months of their schooling, the project's admissions included 12 percent who were married and another 3 percent who were divorced, widowed, or separated. Fully 8 percent of the project's students had children.

In short, the new nursing program had identified an entirely new source of nursing students. Such a development could not fail to please all those who worried about the nursing shortages then haunting the nation's health care system.

When quizzed, the students in the pilot programs said that they had selected the programs first because of the location of the college. These programs allowed them to live at home and commute to school—factors that would naturally have been important considerations for older students with family responsibilities. The length of the program was also a strong attraction, they said. Altogether, 20 percent asserted that they would not have selected a nursing program at all had it not been a part of a community college program.

The withdrawal rates from the programs are more difficult to compare with those from hospital-based programs because of the very different natures of the institutions controlling the two kinds of schools. In the five pilot programs that graduated students by August of 1956, the attrition rate ranged from 20 to 34 percent. But what could not be known was the "stop-out" as opposed to the "drop-out" rates: students in these programs had an option not available to their counterparts in hospital programs—they could transfer from nursing to other majors, and vice versa. Under such circumstances the attrition rate has uncertain meaning.

Follow-up Studies of the Pilot Program Graduates

Follow-up studies of the graduates were imperative, and the CRP staff planned for these from the very beginning of the project. Tracking the performance of graduates began when the first group graduated in 1954. Studies focused on two questions: (1) Did graduates have the ability to qualify for RN licensure? (2) Were they able to perform adequately on the job?

The first question was the focus of a study of six of the seven programs; it traced the performance on licensure examinations of students who had graduated by 1956. (The seventh program had not yet graduated anyone.) Montag found that of the 176 graduates who wrote the licensing examination, 91.7 percent passed on their first attempt. "This compared favorably with the candidates from all nursing programs, whose passing rate was 90.5 percent in 1954 and 91.5 percent in 1955."[23]

In 1964 the results were measured for a much larger sample group. Pilot graduates numbered 562, and other associate degree graduates, 831. Of the 562 pilot program graduates, 477, or 84.9 percent, passed the licensing exam. Of the 831 ADN graduates, 709, or 85.3 percent, passed.[24] These results were in line with those for all other writers in 1964, when 85.7 percent of all writers of the examination passed on the first attempt.

The second question was a more difficult one to deal with initially. Data on job performance were collected from November 1956 to February 1957. Interviews were selected as the measuring device; CRP researchers interviewed project graduates. The interview schedules were designed to elicit information regarding twenty observable behaviors in four general areas of nursing performance: general nursing care, the use of special instruments, clarity and accuracy of oral and written communication, and ability to get along with others. Items concerning a nurse's ability to organize patient care and to perform activities essential to the care unit were added to the interview. Those who were interviewed were asked to rate an ADN graduate's performance, judging whether it was above or below that of graduates of other types of nursing programs who had similar nursing experience.

The sample used in this study included 167 graduates working in twenty-seven hospitals in four states. They represented slightly more than half of the graduates of the pilot programs thus far and about half of the hospitals employing these graduates. It was found that "given some work experience, the graduates of the pilot programs perform the functions of the staff nurse as well as graduates from other programs."[25]

Other conclusions drawn from the studies conducted by the project staff were that

- graduates were able to pass the licensing examinations;
- graduates were able to carry out the functions of the staff nurse;
- the program attracted students;
- the program did become an integral part of the community college;
- the college was able to finance the nursing program just as it did other programs.[26]

Later, in 1964, the questions asked on the original interview schedule were repeated for a much larger sample, with similar results. "An overwhelming percentage of head nurses rated these graduates as good as or better than their counterparts from other nursing programs"[27] — a finding that in the view of some would not apply to all future ADN graduates.

The Impact of the ADN on Nursing Education Growth

The pilot programs conducted under CRP auspices opened the floodgates, or so it seemed at the time. The number of ADN programs grew rapidly, from the original 7 under the project in the 1950s to 677 programs throughout the nation in 1978. The only event like it in the history of nursing education was the explosion in the number of diploma programs that occurred in the early 1900s. Rines reports that from 1952 to 1974 the number of ADN programs doubled about every four years. During one period new programs were opening at the rate of one per week.[28]

The impact on nursing education as a whole was of course significant. When in 1974 the growth began to level off, the new ADN programs constituted 42 percent of all basic education programs in nursing. They were enrolling almost half of all nursing students and graduating 43 percent of the nurses qualified to write state licensing examinations. By 1980 that proportion had grown still more, to 47 percent. Nursing education in colleges and universities now had two branches, the baccalaureate and the associate degree. Moreover, the diploma schools began losing ground; between 1972 and 1978, 202 diploma schools closed.

During the same twenty-five years or so that the ADN program appeared and so firmly established itself in nursing education, the community college also grew rapidly. Clearly, there was a direct relationship between the number of persons choosing community college education and the number choosing ADN programs rather than other kinds of generic nursing programs.

The Impact of the ADN on

Nursing Education

The people who developed the early ADN programs were pioneering individuals who were committed to a new concept in nursing education and willing to take uncharted paths to achieve their goals. In creating the new two-year nursing program, they worked out new curricula and experimented with innovative teaching methods. Many of the ADN educators reported their findings at meetings, in workshops, and in the nursing literature, and as a result they not only influenced one another, they influenced nursing educators in other types of programs. The burst of educational development that marked the 1960s, when the ADN was growing most rapidly, made an especially strong impression on the whole of nursing education, helping to stimulate creative change in many quarters.

The New Nursing Curricula

One of the first things the ADN educators had to do was to negotiate with state boards of nursing to set aside the detailed educational regulations in each state that for years had controlled the curriculum content in nursing schools.[1] Montag recalls that at the outset of the project the CRP had to request that the board of nursing examiners in each state where one of its pilot programs was to be established accede to the CRP's request that all existing regulations with respect to the numbers and sequence of nursing courses be waived.

Because they were unhindered by a tightly defined tradition, the ADN educators were free to create a new educational design. They were free to combine proven educational practices with new ideas and forms. They could test new teaching methods. Virginia Allen remarks that in the early years in ADN education there was little room for individuals who were not willing to challenge traditional practices, experiment with new ones, and take risks. Creating a new model for nursing education required a capacity to think in new ways.

Not all of the innovations of ADN programs were unique to ADN education, but it can be said that the community college environment, where the majority of the ADN programs were located, was conducive to experimentation and innovation. Those who worked on the early programs recall the excitement that pervaded the first years.

A New Method of Curriculum Development. For the first time in the history of nursing, nurse educators were free to write an educational program from scratch. They elected to begin by defining behavioral objectives for their students, a reflection of educational thinking then in vogue. Influenced initially by Tyler's *Basic Principles of Curriculum and Instruction*,[2] and later by Bloom's taxonomy[3] and Mager's work on objectives,[4] ADN faculty spent hours writing objectives in terms of the behavioral changes they wished students to demonstrate. They paid particular attention to objectives dealing with the development of a knowledge base, with skills, and with attitudes—areas commonly referred to as the cognitive, the psychomotor, and the affective. These objectives provided the criteria for selecting all content and experiences for the programs, developing instructional strategies, and evaluating the program components.

What was so innovative about the use of objectives? Until the mid-1950s; most educational objectives were teacher or subject oriented rather than student oriented. Learning activities were prepared and then were carried out, after which students were tested—all without the establishment first of what was to be expected of students who had completed the activities. The structure of a course or program commonly reflected the logical or traditional structure of a given subject matter—or, more often than not, someone's conception of that structure. The ADN programs totally changed this approach, for the entire educational program now was based on clearly delineated objectives regarding student behavior and understanding.

Having worked out these objectives, the ADN faculties then had the means for measuring all the practices and activities that took place in a program. Units of instruction and whole courses could be fine-tuned on the basis of results judged in the light of well-defined goals. Moreover, by using such an approach, the CRP had the means for further studying the role and the behavior of the graduates of the new program, a key factor in its own follow-up studies.

The usefulness of planning a curriculum on the basis of student objectives made an impression on educators in diploma and baccalaureate nursing programs as well, in part because of its success in the ADN programs. Not only that, but the spelling out of the roles and functions of the AD nurse prompted many nurse educators to reexamine and redefine the roles and functions of the graduates of other types of nursing programs.

The Nursing Content. The model provided by the CRP established the assumptions upon which all the early ADN programs were based, even those not established under its auspices. The most basic of these assumptions was that nursing had two clearly differentiated components—the technical and the professional—and that the technical component was the mission of the ADN program. Its nursing content would be organized around common patient problems and nursing interventions to form a comprehensive basis for defining courses. Clinical nursing experiences were to be educationally defined rather than determined by the needs of the moment on a given hospital ward. These experiences were to be planned, directed, controlled, and evaluated by college faculty who would have the freedom to select the health agencies where appropriate experiences for their students would be available. Clinical laboratory experiences were to be credited on the same basis as was any other college laboratory work.

The ADN program would compare with other career-oriented community college programs as to length, total number of credits, and general education requirements, but the nursing component as described in Montag's original research needed further delineation. She had specified that the technical nurse would assist in planning for patient care, giving care, and evaluating it; further, her work made clear that AD nursing would be based on the team approach, as the technical nurse would be working alongside a professional nurse. Clearly, successful performance would require more than just proficiency at individual nursing skills. This was but one of the reasons that Montag emphasized the importance of educational preparation for living "effectively as a person and as a citizen."[5]

Using the behavioral objectives as a framework, the faculties of the earliest programs grouped related nursing content into broad categories. This was the material that would be presented, typically, in one major nursing course required of all nursing students in each of four semesters. Care was taken to organize the content so that students would be provided with continuing opportunities to develop and practice their skills, and then to integrate their experiences with new material as it was presented.

Such a broad-based approach was a radical departure from the traditional nursing curriculum, which was organized around the medical specialties of medicine, surgery, pediatrics, obstetrics, and psychiatry, and which offered in addition separate courses in nursing arts, pharmacology, and diet therapy. It was the students' responsibility to integrate the content of such a curriculum and to apply it to clinical nursing practice. In the new programs those tasks were assumed by the curriculum designers, who built them into the program.

To ensure the progressive development of students' understanding and skills, and to avoid undue repetition, the content of the nursing courses was designed to proceed from simple to complex tasks, from normal to abnormal, from wellness to illness. Interesting frameworks for the ADN curricula emerged: some were based on human growth and development, others on the concept of homeostasis, on the major causes of death, or on major health problems. The broad nursing courses that became standard for ADN programs wove the usual content in pharmacology, diet therapy, nursing, and medical interventions throughout the four semesters in what were often called "curriculum threads." This organizational pattern is still prevalent in ADN programs and has become a design used by other types of nursing programs as well.

Current research in education was not alone in influencing the work of the creators of the first ADN programs; research in nursing care that was being conducted during the 1950s and early 1960s also made its mark. For example, Abdellah's research in patient-centered approaches in nursing was much used by ADN curriculum designers.[6] Abdellah and her colleagues, in an effort to base nursing competence on the nurse's ability to solve key problems presented by patients, engaged in a series of studies that culminated in 1958 with a typology of twenty-one nursing problems and a companion list of the nursing skills needed to solve them. The typology was tested as a curricular approach in three educational settings, one of which was Queens College, New York, where an ADN program was operating under the chairmanship of Ruth V. Matheney. In one description of the program Matheney declared: "Basic nursing education must be patient-centered and to accomplish this, the organization of the curriculum in all its aspects should be such that the patient and his care constitute the goals of learning."[7]

The ADN Movement and Educational Methodology

The first associate degree faculties were also pioneers in bringing new methods of instruction and evaluation to nursing education. The national attention they received from their workshops and forums, and the publications that issued from those meetings, brought their innovations to the attention of nursing faculties everywhere.

One of the new techniques was the use of the clinical conference in the laboratory component of the nursing program. The conferences provided a means for directing the student's learning in clinical settings. The preconference enabled students and faculty to discuss the learning objectives of a planned clinical experience. Students were assigned patients and guided in planning and organizing data collection and patient care. The postconference provided the opportunity for students to describe their experiences, ask questions, clarify the relationship between theory and practice on the basis of the immediate experience, and thus increase their understanding of the nurse's role. As experience mounts, the pre- and postconferences become occasions for identifying the commonalities of care among diverse assignments and thus for forming generalizations about and guidelines for nursing interventions. Of equal importance, of course, was the fact that such conferences provided students with the opportunity to share their emotional experiences and to gain peer support.[8]

ADN educators were also innovative in the way they organized clinical assignments. The correlation of nursing theory and practice required the careful selection of patients for students' clinical experiences. Faculty members often face a shortage of appropriate cases for given learning objectives. Moreover, they are responsible not only to the student for educational results but also to both student and patient for maintaining safe student-teacher ratios. Maura Carroll introduced a method of clinical assignment that addressed these complex problems by assigning several students to the same patient during the same laboratory period. In her approach, which she tested and found effective and which many ADN programs adopted for testing and use in their own settings, the three students assigned to one patient had separate roles: one was the doer, one the observer, and the third the information gatherer. The doer administered the nursing care and recorded pertinent patient information; the observer watched both the doer and the patient's reactions, as well as all aspects of the environment, to later report to the rest of the team; the information gatherer served as a resource for the doer by becoming thoroughly acquainted with the patient's record. This method, now known as "multiple assignment," has been implemented with many variations in ADN and other programs; the number of students assigned to a patient may be any number from two to five, but all variants have the virtue of facilitating the correlation of theory to practice, increasing the number of students one instructor can manage in a clinical situation, and perhaps most importantly, of providing students with repeated experience as members of a team.[9]

Another instructional innovation experimented with by the early ADN faculty members was programmed instruction. In 1963 Marie Seedor published her research on its use in community college nursing programs, describing its purpose as twofold: "to develop programmed material and to determine whether or not nursing students could learn" by this means.[10] ADN faculty members were drawn to this method because of its usefulness for students as heterogeneous as ADN student bodies tend to be. Programmed instruction is self-paced, actively involves the student, and provides immediate feedback and evaluation. Seedor chose asepsis as the subject for programming that she tested using students from Bronx Community College, New York, and Dutchess Community College, New York. Her success encouraged ADN faculty members everywhere to develop their own materials, use commercially prepared packages, or combine the two to design instruction for their own students.

Programmed instruction, though, was not the only means for providing students with the autonomy of self-paced learning and immediate feedback. In 1964 Samuel Postlethwait, a professor at Purdue University, described the design of his biology course to ADN educators attending a national conference, who reacted with great excitement. Postlethwait combined group sessions with the use of audiovisual materials, printed materials, and laboratory experiences in such a way as to create a learning center where students could study independently, pace their own learning, and receive individualized instruction and feedback from faculty.[11] ADN educators adopted this idea for audio-tutorial systems for independent study in the belief that it would be particularly appropriate for students from diverse backgrounds.

Crystal Lange became known for her application of Postlethwait's principles to the teaching of nursing techniques at Delta College in Michigan. She established a learning laboratory where she used a multisensory approach to help students perfect their skills before performing them in a clinical setting.[12] Postlethwait's methods were adopted by many ADN programs, and campus learning laboratories mushroomed as the community colleges and ADN programs continued to flourish through the 1960s. The laboratories varied in the sophistication of their use of new technologies, but all were based on the same educational principles.

From 1962 to 1965 the nursing program at Bronx Community College explored the feasibility of using closed-circuit television for clinical instruction, which the faculty put into use for the first time in 1965. A faculty member was able to observe and instruct fifteen students in a single laboratory session by using television cameras, monitors, and a two-way communication system. It was found that the instructor-student contact was eight times greater with the use of the television technology than without.[13]

The learning centers in many ADN schools became the settings for evaluating clinical skills. The nursing faculty at Orange County Community College, New York, experimented with what was called the "walk-around laboratory practical examination." Students moved from station to station, each of which posed a nursing problem that the student could solve only by synthesizing theoretical knowledge and applying nursing principles. The solutions required the student to observe closely, manipulate equipment, and make judgments. The system placed each student taking the examination in the same situation with the same variables, thereby making it possible to systematically evaluate students' behavioral achievements.[14]

Before long, faculties had incorporated such laboratory performance examinations into the standard ADN program, making the exams an integral part of the nursing courses. Simulated patient situations were created that paralleled didactic teaching and that required students to integrate what they had learned and to put it into action. Allen recalls one such examination, designed to test students' knowledge of environmental hazards. As each student left the station, with answers recorded, the faculty found that the hazards had also been carefully corrected. They had to hastily reset the stage before the next student could enter the station!

The identification of "critical elements" used for evaluating nursing performance was another innovation adopted early on by many ADN educators, and it, too, soon became a common means of evaluating students using the campus laboratory. At first, checklists for the evaluation of specific nursing skills were developed, listing satisfactory and unsatisfactory behaviors. Eventually the method was refined, as faculty members became more sophisticated in identifying critical requirements, defined as those behaviors that must be demonstrated by a student if performance of a skill is to be judged safe. Undoubtedly, the best example of the use of critical elements to evaluate specific skills is the performance-in-nursing examination of the New York Regents External Degree Nursing Program, developed first for associate degree applicants for a degree. Many publications now in the literature describe the key concepts for developing and implementing performance examinations.[15]

Innovative methods of teaching and evaluation like those described here are now in wide use throughout all of nursing education. They were developed first and most fully in the early ADN programs because of their need to meet the special challenge posed by the heterogeneity of their students. The methods that were based on self-directed and self-paced learning were the most distinctive of the methods that were introduced into basic nursing education by the ADN program pioneers. Although they contributed most directly to program goals unique to ADN education, even these techniques for independent study have proven to be useful in other programs as well.

The W. K. Kellogg Foundation and the

Four-State Project

By the mid-1950s, even before the CRP had been completed, many observers were coming to believe that the two-year associate degree program might provide the best solution to the nursing shortage. Three-year hospital-based programs had shown a slow but steady decline. In 1951 diploma programs had numbered 1,065, or 84 percent of all programs, but during the next ten years their number dropped precipitously, to 883, with further drops yet to come.[1] In the meantime, two-year associate degree programs were flourishing in the community colleges, and their growth was likely to be even more rapid in years to come. In 1957 four states—California, Florida, New York, and Texas—were developing proposals for statewide action on behalf of ADN education. It was no accident that the community college movement was strong in all of these states.

In 1957 Dr. Mildred Tuttle, director of the W. K. Kellogg Foundation's Division of Nursing, was being advised by the Nursing Advisory Committee, which was made up almost entirely of new members. The one veteran was Marian Sheahan, at this time the associate director of the NLN. The newcomers to the foundation's advisory group were Dr. Mildred Newton, dean of the School of Nursing of Ohio State University; Dr. Mildred Montag, at this time directing the ongoing work of the CRP; and Dr. Marguerite Kakosh, most recently director of nursing studies with the VA hospital system.[2]

At the first meeting of the new group, 22, 23, and 24 August 1957, Montag summarized her findings to date in the CRP's evaluation of the development of ADN education. These conclusions, which were to be reported in a publication due to be issued early in 1958, were as follows:

–it was possible to prepare a graduate nurse in the community college to carry on functions commonly associated with the graduate of the traditional hospital-based school of nursing.

–it was possible to make the nursing program an integral part of the junior college with the same administrative structure as any other program in the college.

–the program was proving to be attractive to students, especially to older students. Twenty percent [probably too low an estimate] of all students in the ADN programs chose nursing because the program was located in a junior college.

–the withdrawal rates from ADN programs were lower than in other nursing programs.

–the curriculum included the same credits for classroom and laboratory practice, the same admissions standards, and the same standards for faculty qualifications and salaries as other programs in the college.

–finally, the satisfaction of both faculty and students in the new programs was high.[3]

After discussing Montag's report, the committee suggested the following plan of action to the foundation:

1. Select one or more states as sites and then develop for each a state plan listing the number of junior colleges and community resources. Use this information to determine the programs needed and then identify those colleges that best meet established criteria for selection as sites for new ADN programs. [In all likelihood, the criteria used by the CRP under Montag's direction were what the committee had in mind.]

2. Provide consultation to the colleges by teams of experts whose expertise would cover junior college education and nursing education. NLN would supply one team.

3. Provide state and regional work conferences to initiate and train all persons who would be involved in developing and running the junior college nursing programs.

4. Develop instructional materials "illustrating the best practices of nursing programs in the CRP pilot schools to be used by faculty developing new programs and by hospital-based programs seeking to improve their curricula."

5. Select and prepare teachers for junior college nursing programs, pos-

sibly using teacher training programs available in Texas, in California, and at Teachers College, Columbia University.[4]

Two themes dominated the advisory committee's related discussion of ways to attract more young women into nursing: the need to develop a new curricular pattern that would provide a broader preparation than those "currently in vogue" and the need to prepare more and better teachers in nursing. The latter was the first priority in nursing, in the opinion of the committee, which believed that current fellowship assistance was inadequate, unable to supply the numbers needed. (The program set up by Congress in 1955 had awarded fewer than one hundred fellowships annually, for example.) Particularly urgent was the need to improve the quality of practice teaching and to identify and document the best practices in teacher training in nursing.[5]

The advisory committee met again on 21–22 November 1957, and once again it devoted a considerable portion of its time to discussing the new associate degree program in nursing. Sheahan reported that the NLN had been considering "the problem of nursing personnel needs in relation to population trends and has estimated that a forty percent increase in the number of nurses will be required to meet minimum needs in 1970, and a sixty percent increase will be necessary if the optimum goal of 350 nurses per 100,000 population is to be reached." Committee members noted that the nation's nursing schools were annually graduating 29,000 students and that the number needed by 1970 was 48,000. Sheahan pointed out the urgent need for additional programs in basic nursing in the far West and in the South, if minimum goals were to be reached by 1970. Montag noted the phenomenal growth of junior colleges in California and their interest in developing nursing programs. Both Sheahan and Montag stressed the need for good consultation services to junior colleges that were establishing new nursing programs. The consensus of the advisory committee was that the "greatest bottleneck to the success of such programs is the complete lack of prepared faculty for such programs."[6]

The committee once again endorsed the foundation's interest in further exploring the potential of the ADN programs and suggested that it initiate a program similar to the one it had recently funded in practical nurse education in five southern states. That program had awarded grants to state departments of education for reallocation to local junior college programs, had provided a state or regional consultant to communities and colleges that were opening programs, and had provided pre-service and in-service training for the faculties of junior college programs. A like program to prepare nurses at the master's level for teaching in junior college programs, the committee suggested, would assist selected universities. The program would orient students to the philosophy, objectives, organization, and administration of junior colleges, assist them in the planning of appropriate curricula, provide field experience in junior colleges and community agencies, provide consultation to faculties of junior colleges located near the universities participating in the program, and provide in-service education for those same faculties.

The committee further suggested starting in one state to obtain experience. California was put forward as the state having the most experience and "the greatest problems." The first step, they thought, might be an informal conference with representatives from the state department of education, followed by a similar meeting with representatives of junior colleges and nursing organizations.[7]

The next few years saw continued explosive growth in junior college education: by 1960, 521 two-year colleges were claiming an enrollment of 451,000 students. During this period, although approximately half of these schools were publicly controlled, they accounted for most of the total junior college enrollment. By 1958, forty-eight nursing programs had been instituted in junior colleges.[8] Kellogg officials willingly provided funds to help finance the cost of state-level meetings to plan more coherent growth and development for nursing education in these institutions.

California was indeed the site of the earliest conference to plan a statewide program. Held 5 and 6 June 1958, it was conducted under the leadership of the California Junior College Association (CJCA), which invited about twenty leaders in nursing and education to help draft a statewide plan to develop and improve ADN programs. Fourteen people representing the junior colleges, the CJCA, the state department of education, state nursing organizations, and the University of California at Los Angeles prepared a plan that emphasized four points: they believed that a successful plan depended on the availability of adequate consulting services, careful evaluation of progress, assistance to individual schools in securing staff, and the provision for pre- and in-service education for staff.[9] A second and longer conference was held in California a few months later. From 23 June through 11 July 1958, participants met to discuss the administration, organization, curriculum, and instructional methods of associate degree nursing education. Eleven of the participants were from states other than California.[10]

Kellogg's advisory committee in nursing met again on 30 June and 1 July 1958, and reviewed a funding request from the CJCA for a five-year grant to assist with the strengthening of existing ADN programs in California and the development of new programs. The proposal suggested (1) the establishment of a pre-service program at the University of California at Los Angeles to prepare faculty, (2) a consultation program for junior college administrators and nursing directors and faculty of existing nursing programs, and (3) an in-service educational program for faculty members responsible for the existing programs. Because the state board of nursing had only temporarily approved the ADN programs, plans for an evaluation phase of the project were included.[11]

The committee again endorsed the placement of a project in the state of California and also identified other states as possible project sites: Texas, Florida, New York, Pennsylvania, Illinois, Michigan, and Mississippi. Once again the areas it suggested for program development were these:

1. a graduate program to prepare teachers and directors;
2. continuing education for the faculty members of existing ADN programs;
3. consultation services;
4. additional pilot programs to serve as demonstration centers to be used for the orientation of new faculty and as practice-teaching sites for graduate students;
5. planning activities to precede the start-up dates of new programs.[12]

The advisory committee again recommended fellowships for nursing students interested in preparing to direct or teach in junior college programs. They pointed out that the fellowships and traineeships then available from both private and public sources provided no concentration on any one type of school or program. "It was felt that, since junior college programs [were] new, and to some nurses, 'controversial,' fellowships would provide a recruitment incentive to nurses who might become interested in participating in a new and challenging movement in basic nurse education."[13]

In the meantime, project planning in Texas was launched, under the leadership of the University of Texas. An initial meeting was held in Austin 7–8 August 1958, attended by persons representing the Texas League for Nursing, the Texas Graduate Nurses' Association, the state board of nursing, various hospitals, the University of Texas School of Nursing, the junior college division of the state department of education, a number of junior colleges, and two consultants from other states who were familiar with nursing programs in junior colleges. Discussions provided the twenty or so people attending the meeting with a better understanding of the associate degree program and also provided planners with an opportunity to sound out the various organizations about their positions regarding the expansion of ADN programs in the state. The occasion made it possible for planners in Texas to determine the state's readiness for expansion of the ADN idea. The consensus was that careful planning would be needed and that a slow approach to developing a statewide plan was advisable. In fact, a second conference was recommended, to involve a larger number of people.[14] Planning was held up temporarily, pending the outcome of new nursing legislation that would permit the state board of nursing to approve a nursing program of only two calendar years. When that law was finally passed in April 1959, the subcommittee resumed work on a statewide plan.

Kellogg's officers and consultants continued to focus attention on the coming shortages of nurses and the inability of existing educational facilities to meet the need. As Mildred Tuttle later described the problem to the board of trustees, in June 1959, "our present 944 hospital schools of nursing are virtually filled to capacity and . . . most of our 167 college and university schools of nursing can admit relatively few additional students." However, only a small proportion of the nation's 667 community and junior colleges had established nursing programs; clearly, "within this latter group lay the greatest potential for the preparation of increased numbers of nursing personnel." The foundation's director of nursing programs declared that she "looked to the associate degree programs in nursing in our junior and community colleges as the most promising development on the nursing horizon today."[15]

During the fall, winter, and spring of 1958–1959 the foundation continued to assemble the components of a major new program that would be focused on the preparation of nurses at the pre-service level—that is, in basic nursing education. A third state, New York, entered the picture in February 1959, when the commissioner of education of the University of the State of New York (an administrative body, not a school, despite its name), determined to develop a statewide plan for New York.

A small conference was called to plan the development of ADN programs in the state. Persons to be invited to this meeting would include representatives of Teachers College, Columbia University (home of the CRP), the State University of New York, and the state department of education, which included the state board of nursing. Kellogg agreed to fund the conference, whose purpose was to design a statewide plan for developing ADN programs in junior colleges.

Florida faced a unique situation: during the 1950s the state's population showed a nearly 50 percent increase, as roughly 5,000 new residents moved in every week. New hospitals were being built at a furious pace; the number of hospital beds increased by 2,500 between 1951 and 1957, and another 1,000 were scheduled to open in 1959. Yet only 4 percent of the women high school graduates were entering nursing in Florida, a rate well below the national average of 7 percent. Compounding the problem was the concentration of the existing nurse pool in a few urban areas.[16] Florida's version of the nursing shortage threatened to be an acute one.

Anticipating the problem, the Florida legislature in 1955 established the Community College Council and charged it with the responsibility for making long-range plans for junior college expansion in Florida. The keystone of the plan that the council presented to the Florida State Board of Education was its coverage of the entire state; 99 percent of the population would live within commuting distance of a public junior college. The state's junior colleges indeed grew rapidly, as the plan was put into action. By 1959, ten areas that were operating junior colleges represented 29 percent of the state population; about 9,000 students were enrolled in junior colleges by the fall of 1958. The junior college students represented 19 percent of all college students in the state, 33 percent of all freshmen.[17]

Growth was rapid but coherent, thanks in part to the work of the Interorganization Committee, which long preceded the Kellogg Foundation's involvement in the state's ADN programs. The committee, formed in the early 1950s, consisted of three representatives of the state board of nursing and three from junior colleges, as well as Dr. Leon Henderson of the University of Florida, Dr. Henry Ashmore of Pensacola Junior College, and Dr. James Wattenbarger of the state department of education. They issued a report that was widely distributed and much discussed.[18] The principles articulated early on in Florida were repeated in other states. Prominent among them were these ideas:

1. Community colleges can best aid nursing education by developing recruitment programs, by using good guidance and counseling procedures, and by developing programs of nursing education that resemble other programs in the community college.

2. The nursing education program developed in the community college should be tailored to meet the requirements of educating nurses and not merely attempt to fit the education of nurses into some preconceived number of months.

3. The community college should work very closely with the state board of nursing and with the state department of education to develop the curriculum.

4. The program for nursing education in the community college should be designed as an associate degree program. It should not be developed as a preparatory program for two additional years leading to a bachelor's degree.

5. Community colleges might also develop programs for training practical nurses, but these should be entirely separate from the ADN program.

6. The state board of nursing should help the state department of education to determine whether a community has enough clinical services available to permit a program for nursing education to be organized in a particular community college.

7. Community college nursing education should not be designed to replace the existing hospital programs of nursing education.

8. Finally, research must be conducted to determine how much time and what skills are needed in the education of the nurse, particularly, to evaluate the amount of time that is now spent in hospital-based diploma programs.[19]

Given the high level of interest in junior and community college development in Florida, it is no surprise that the state law in the late 1950s regarding the minimum length of pre-service nursing programs made it possible for associate degree graduates to write the state licensing examination.

Florida's proposals were added to those from New York and from the planning conferences held earlier in Texas and California. Thus, planners from all four states helped to design the master plan for a long-term four-state project in ADN educational development. The planning conferences had achieved much beyond their immediate task of helping to draft the overall proposal for the four-state project. They oriented people in these states to plans and issues that would be critical to AD education later on, and they provided the occasion for soliciting wider support for the new ADN programs.

Kellogg's focus on ADN education reflected not only its concern that the existing educational system could not meet the increasing demand for nurses but also its conviction that the CRP directed by Montag at Columbia had been successful. In the annual report to the foundation of nursing program activity as of May 1959, Tuttle described the CRP's pilot programs this way:

1. Objectives of the nursing program were consistent with the over-all objectives of the college and were acceptable [to] the nursing profession.
2. The college controlled the entire program and assumed the entire financial responsibility for it.
3. The nursing faculty were employed by the college and had equal status with other college faculty.
4. The nursing students had the same status as the college students in other fields of study.
5. The program included general education as well as nursing education.
6. Nursing courses were fewer in number, but broader in scope than in the traditional three-year program.
7. Nursing practice was selected in terms of the students' learning needs, and repetitive practice was reduced to a minimum.
8. Learning experiences were centered on patients' needs and on the essential nursing activities.[20]

Tuttle further explained that the foundation's interest in the ADN programs was based on the fact that "such programs . . . attract an additional number of young people into the field of nursing for the following reasons: students could live at home and go to school; the programs were within the financial grasp of the majority of students; and the curriculum represented a new and challenging approach to learning the basic principles and practice of nursing."[21]

The total 1958–1959 appropriation by Kellogg in support of ADN education in four states amounted to $1,569,000.[22] This sum does not include the funds the foundation provided for the planning conferences in California, Texas, New York, and Florida. In addition, Kellogg officials awarded similar but separate grants to a statewide program in Illinois, to the Chicago Board of Education for ADN development in the metropolitan area, and to Purdue University and the University of Kentucky to "assist them in instituting junior college nursing in their respective spheres of influence." The foundation's assistance overall to ADN education at this juncture thus totaled more than $3 million.[23]

The four-state project, designed to promote planned statewide growth of ADN programs in Florida, Texas, New York, and California, was the centerpiece of Kellogg's overall intention to help education meet the nation's need for more nurses. The consensus that emerged from the planning was that the foundation's aid should emphasize (1) faculty preparation, (2) continuing education, (3) consultation services, (4) demonstration centers, (5) planning and evaluation of programs and graduates, and (6) in-service programs for employing agencies. Because it was generally recognized that finding teachers for the new program was going to be an especially difficult problem—not only were qualified nursing instructors generally in short supply, but those prepared to teach in the new technical program were extremely rare—much of the project was focused on ADN faculty development. The project also included plans to establish teacher-preparation programs in the state universities of the four funded states.[24]

On 4 and 5 June 1959, the Nursing Advisory Committee once again met with Tuttle to review foundation work in nursing. Faye Abdellah, Mildred Newton, Mildred Montag, and Rozella Schlotfeldt discussed the issues that they hoped the foundation's nursing programs would address. Two committee members were new: Schlotfeldt was on the nursing faculty of Wayne State University and Abdellah was with the U.S. Public Health Service.

The advisory committee deliberated, knowing all too well the difficulties nursing education was facing because of the nursing shortage, which was now reaching a crisis state. In 1958 there were 430,000 RNs in the United States, but some experts were saying that by 1970 the nation would need 600,000 to maintain health services at the 1958 level. To supply that need, nursing schools, which in 1956 had admitted 45,255 students, would by some estimates have to be attracting at least 75,000 each year by 1970, nearly twice as many. The schools graduated 29,933 nurses in 1956–1957; by 1970 some officials believed they would have to graduate 48,000 to meet the nation's needs.[25] There was

little time to spare, and the task seemed to be enormous; careful planning and rapid growth would both be needed—a tall order.

Issues that would continue to plague ADN education were raised
at this meeting. Abdellah and Schlotfeldt questioned whether the
instructional programs for junior college nursing schools were in fact
different from those that had been used in better university schools of
nursing for some time. They also questioned the advisability of establishing an entirely new program at the graduate level to prepare faculty
specifically for ADN education. Montag and Newton believed that
specific preparation for teaching in junior college programs was needed.
All the members agreed, however, that all students in pre-service programs to prepare nurses for faculty positions, regardless of the type of
college, should take "core courses," including those in a clinical specialty and those focused on the teaching of that specialty to undergrad-
uates. They also agreed that the ADN programs should be terminal and
that "the graduate should be classified as a semi-professional worker in
the nursing services."[26]

The California Projects. In its California portion, the four-state project mounted a three-pronged attack on the problems of rapid ADN development. The state's department of education assumed responsibility
for coordinating ADN growth in the state by offering consulting services to schools that had or were planning to open two-year nursing
programs, by assembling and disseminating all available information
regarding the ADN and its development in the state, and by conducting
status and evaluation studies of ongoing ADN programs. In accordance
with the overall objectives of the four-state project, the University of
California in Los Angeles conducted two instructional programs, one a
pre-service program for nurses who planned to teach in ADN programs
and the other an in-service program for current faculty. The direct grant
to Los Angeles Valley College supported the creation of a curriculum
demonstration center for the state's ADN schools.[27]

California's entry into ADN education had been energetic and swift,
in no small part because the state's junior colleges had been well established beginning in the early 1900s (see chapter 3 for details). By 1959,
in fact, there were thirteen two-year nursing programs in the state, and
seven more were but one year away from admitting their first students.[28]
All three facets of the California project faced enormous task loads in
the face of such growth.

The state was more forward-looking than many in its laws regarding the new two-year program. The California legislature authorized the state board of nursing to accredit two-year courses for a five-year provisional period. Just how important the measure was is revealed in the results of a study conducted by the chairman of one ADN program in California. Her national survey of licensing laws indicated that at the end of the 1950s nine of the fifty states did not license the graduates of nursing programs only two years long, though three of the nine were considering liberalizing their laws. Thirty-two states placed no barriers before two-year nursing graduates, who could write the state exam along with the graduates of other, longer programs and earn licensure if they passed the exam. Two states allowed the two-year programs but had written into state law requirements specifying the content that two-year curricula should include. Four states licensed two-year graduates on an individual basis, and three would do so only if the applicant could present an employer's statement of competence.[29] Obviously, revision of state laws throughout the nation would play an essential role in ADN growth.

Despite the strong head start that ADN education enjoyed in California, the demonstration center at Los Angeles Valley College in Van Nuys identified certain problems. Most important, the nursing and hospital community was not uniformly ready to accept the new program. Other, more minor problems included the discovery that students in the programs exhibited attention problems attributed to fatigue and stress, clinical specialty teaching was not possible for faculty, and additional teacher time was used to fill in material in pharmacology that had been integrated into the overall curricular content. Also, students complained of their inability to master manual skills under the program as it was structured.[30]

Most of these problems and complaints were not unique to the AD program. Some students also noted their inability to learn their way around the college and often participated little in college activities because of their heavy clinical loads. The majority of the students in the project were single (61–65 percent), and many (40 percent) had previous experience in junior and senior colleges. Two-thirds of the students would have chosen the AD program even if a hospital-based or a baccalaureate program had been readily available.

From 1960 to 1964, as a result of project activities and the pool of California students, faculty, and institutions influenced by the project's work, the number of associate degree programs in the state almost doubled (from sixteen to thirty) and the number of students enrolled grew from 913 to 2,312.

The Florida Projects. Before 1959 in Florida there were but two junior colleges offering ADN programs, Pensacola Junior College and St. Petersburg Junior College. But in 1959–1960 a third ADN program was established, at West Palm Beach, and plans for yet others were being made. The Kellogg Foundation's five-year commitment to the state under the four-state project came at an opportune time.

The part of the Florida project that was centered in the state's education department emphasized the needs of schools that were planning new ADN programs slated to open shortly. The department of education would employ two consultants who would assist selected colleges during the planning year preceding the opening of a new ADN program.

Other parts of the project included in-service education for the persons who would be teaching or employing the new ADN students and graduates, a demonstration center for ADN curriculum development, and a teacher training program based at the University of Florida. Here, as in the other project states, faculty development was a need receiving much attention. Efforts at the University of Florida's College of Nursing were directed first toward the preparation of faculty for new junior college nursing schools. Plans were that the college of nursing faculty would work closely with faculty from the colleges of education, business administration, arts and sciences, and graduate schools to develop a curriculum in nursing at the master's level. No master's in nursing program then existed in the state, and it was generally believed that such a program was a cornerstone in the development of sound ADN programs.

The Florida project was overseen by an advisory committee that met twice a year to review work, recommend program improvements, and develop long-range recommendations for ADN programs in the state. The committee included representatives of the state board of nursing, the state hospital and medical associations, the Florida League for Nursing, the Florida Nurses' Association, the University of Florida College of Education, the University of Florida School of Nursing, Florida State University, the Practical Nurse Association, the State Association of Junior Colleges, the State Advisory Council on Education, and the Junior College Curriculum Center. It was constituted so as to muster the broadest possible support for the new program. An executive committee that met six times a year established policy for the overall program for the state under the four-state project; it directed program activities and reported to the advisory committee.[31]

The Florida projects' results were similar to those in California. The number of associate degree programs more than tripled (from three to ten), and the number of enrollments grew from 203 to 644.

The New York Projects. In 1958 the Research Office of the State Department of Education, University of the State of New York, completed a report of a study by a committee known as the Nurse Resources Study Group.[32] The committee identified the community college as the most flexible of all institutions of higher education and highlighted the significance of its contribution, the terminal technical curricula leading to nursing occupations. The report asserted that the community college was in a unique position to prepare much-needed nursing personnel and in so doing also find new patterns of nursing education. Obviously, the climate in New York was right for rapid development of the ADN idea.

The New York projects had four facets, which resembled those in Florida and California. One, centered at Teachers College, Columbia University, would prepare ADN teachers. A second would assist selected colleges during the planning year preceding the formal opening of a new ADN program. Consulting services from a central source and available statewide would be provided, and in-service education programs for faculty and staff of concerned agencies would be created and executed. A curriculum center to establish priorities for curriculum development and create teaching materials and curriculum guides would be based at Bronx Community College, which would also be used to provide graduate students in the Teachers College program student-teaching opportunities.

In December 1959 the project assembled the directors of the state's six ADN programs; they met in a workshop to discuss a number of issues of concern to ADN educators: the integration of general education with nursing education, student evaluation and counseling, and follow-up studies of ADN graduates. The project sponsored a special study group that prepared a set of guidelines for colleges wishing to survey hospitals and other community facilities that might provide laboratory experience for ADN students. Statewide planning continued under project aegis; the focus was on the geographical distribution of junior colleges, hospitals, and other clinical facilities throughout the state.

The graduate faculty at Teachers College developed a full-year master's program for the initial preparation of teachers for ADN programs. The program focuses included the purpose, organization, and curriculum of junior colleges; the techniques of teaching nursing; and the advanced study of specialized nursing practice. The program included courses from those offered all students preparing for educational positions in higher education. In 1959 and 1960 seventeen students were enrolled in the new master's program, and six others in nursing were seeking doctoral degrees.

The faculty and students in the new program at Teachers College saw quickly how urgent the need was for instructional materials for the new ADN curriculum. They were in a unique position to develop, test, and evaluate such materials. As a consequence, the faculty was able to provide consulting services to others on matters concerning curriculum development. Much of this pioneering work reached print as well, in which form it could make an even wider impact on ADN development throughout the nation.[33]

The New York project was administered by the State Advisory Committee and the Coordinating Council, which was the policy-making group. Dr. Robert Kinsinger, formerly with the NLN, served the project as the specialist in junior college education. In early 1960 Mary Topalis, formerly director of the nursing program at Fairleigh Dickinson University in New Jersey, joined the project as staff specialist in nursing education. Fairleigh Dickinson was the site of one of the earliest schools to participate in the CRP, based at Teachers College.[34]

The results in New York resembled those in the other states. The number of associate degree programs grew from four to fifteen, the number of students enrolled grew from 195 to 816, and the number of faculty prepared far exceeded those of other projects. The high number reflected the head start New York possessed by virtue of its being the site of the CRP.

The Texas Projects. In 1959 Texas ranked second in the country in the number of its junior colleges—46 were operating when the Kellogg project began. Only California boasted more two-year colleges. At the same time Texas was experiencing an acute shortage of nurses; there were 128 nurses for every 100,000 population, when 268 were needed to bring the state up to par with the national average.[35] In 1957 the state's eight baccalaureate programs graduated only 177 nurses and the hospital programs numbered only 600—far short of the state's needs. Moreover, all the existing schools were located in urban areas. Under the circumstances, development of ADN programs looked promising: 34 of the 46 junior colleges were publicly financed, and their tuitions were affordable to many students who could not consider the more expensive programs in nursing then available.

The University of Texas had taken the lead in promoting the growth of junior colleges in the state, including the development of ADN programs. Even before the Kellogg Foundation expressed an interest in ADN development in the state, Texas had an advisory committee working on a statewide plan. Once the Kellogg project was under way, a steering committee from this group was appointed; its purpose was to select colleges to participate in the four-state project. Members were Marjorie Bartholf, dean of the University of Texas School of Nursing; Ruth McFarland, nurse consultant to the junior college project; and two representatives of the university College of Education, Dr. C. C. Colvert and Dr. James Reynolds. Ultimately, this committee became the official body administering the project, formulating its policies and making decisions regarding the overall program.[36]

The purposes of the Kellogg commitment to the University of Texas were essentially the same as those for the other three states: to establish pilot ADN programs in three junior colleges, to offer master's-level education for the preparation of AD faculty, to conduct summer workshops for teachers in ADN programs, and to establish a demonstration center for curriculum development.[37] The first junior college selected to participate was Odessa Community College in Odessa, Texas. The project also located its demonstration center at Odessa College. Later, two other ADN programs were established with Kellogg assistance: one at Texarkana and the other at San Jacinto. One workshop was held; in the summer of 1962 a program entitled "Nursing Education in Junior Colleges" drew thirty-eight people interested in the possibility of teaching in ADN programs. No students were ever enrolled in the university program to prepare nursing faculty for associate degree programs.

On the whole, the Texas projects did not enjoy the immediate success that similar projects had in the other three states. Assessments of the programs varied; the reasons offered in evaluations to explain the disappointing initial results included the following. First, cost proved to be a barrier. Administrators could not see why nursing could not be like any other collegiate program with respect to student-teacher ratios, a complaint that was to surface elsewhere later on. Second, the sheer size of the state proved to be a factor; travel distances and the difficulty of maintaining direct communications in the face of these distances proved to be a crippling problem. Odessa, for instance, was so isolated that it never actually functioned as a demonstration center, as planned.[38] A third source of difficulty seemed to be the state board of nursing. To quote the report to the foundation trustees of 1963, when Kellogg funds for the program were terminated, "the major inhibitory factor was the attitude of the State Board of Nursing toward the program and the increasing number of requirements of the Board which were imposed upon the junior colleges" having ADN programs.[39] The length of the programs, the course content, and the clinical hours proved to be sticking points. A fourth problem was the lack of interest in the ADN as a terminal program; state financial support was directed more to the first two years of a four-year program. Fifth, leadership was not forthcoming from the Texas Education Agency or the state junior college association.

Despite these immediate problems, the long-term effects of the effort were most gratifying. The ADN idea had been planted, and it grew as the years passed. The five years of the four-state project in Texas had proven insufficient time to measure lasting effects. By 1983 Texas had established forty ADN programs throughout the state, and 5,479 students were pursuing the ADN degree. Texas by the 1980s was considered a leader in the ADN movement.

The Federal Government Lends a Hand

The promotion of the ADN program by the CRP and the four-state project demonstrated nationally that there were sound reasons for establishing nursing programs in America's community colleges. ADN programs were located within the general system of the nation's higher education, a goal long desired by nursing reformers; they graduated nurses competent to perform within the existing health care system; and they provided good solutions to the nursing shortage. The momentum established by the CRP and the four-state project was soon to be stepped up by federal assistance to the students, the faculty, and the college, which became available to ADN programs during the 1960s.

Health Care Expansion and the Nursing Shortage

The American health care system expanded rapidly after the end of World War II; growth was especially vigorous after 1952. Selected statistics suggest how very great the system's expansion was. In 1945 the nation was spending just under $1 billion annually on its short-term nonfederal hospitals, that is to say, its general hospitals; sixteen years later that expenditure had grown to five times that amount.[1] The nation's spending on health care rose as well: in terms of 1985 dollars, Americans were spending $318 per capita on health care in 1948, $588 in 1962—nearly twice as much. During the same period the percentage of the gross national product devoted to health care had risen, from 4.1 to 5.6 percent.[2] In 1961 the health system payroll was seven times what it had been just after the war.[3] From 1950 to 1960 the health service work force grew at a rate of 54 percent.[4] The ratio of health care personnel to patients changed as new treatment modalities were developed and the use of nursing assistants expanded: in 1945 there were 155 workers per patient, but in 1961 there were 226.[5]

The growth of the health care system exerted intense pressures on nursing during the first fifteen years after the war. The ranks of registered nurses did not expand at anywhere near the same rate as the system as a whole. Much more growth was visible among licensed practical nurses (LPNs) and nursing aides, a matter of concern that would be voiced by the surgeon general's nursing consultants later on. The number of aides in general hospitals roughly equaled the number of RNs in 1961, and in long-term hospitals there were four times as many aides as nurses. Unit managers and ward secretaries—additional auxiliary personnel—were also employed to help lighten the workload. As the hospitals struggled to meet the growing shortage of registered nurses, plans for grouping patients according to their nursing and medical needs were tried, and specialty and self-care units were developed, which ironically only intensified the shortage.

Intensive care units (ICUs) were being established in hospital after hospital, most of them devoted to a subspecialty area. Coronary care, neurological, and renal units were the most common of these, plus units devoted to the care of infection-prone patients. Nurses were found to be the "most important factor in the unit" in such settings, and their staff-to-patient ratios were much higher than in any other location in the hospital. When in 1967 the Division of Nursing provided funds to Presbyterian Hospital in Philadelphia to establish a coronary care unit, it was determined that 250 similar units had been set up elsewhere in the country.[6]

The postwar emphasis on marriage and family also played an important part in the number of nurses wanting to work, and during the 1950s and into the early 1960s increasing numbers of young women were choosing early marriage and child-rearing over careers. From 1890 to 1962 the median age of marriage for women dropped steadily, from 22 to 20.3, and in 1962, three-quarters of a million young women married between the ages of fourteen and nineteen. In 1900, two of every three women married at some time during their lives, but in 1962 the proportion had risen to four of five. The birth rate had also risen: in 1960 there were 488 children under the age of five for every 1,000 women; 291 would have been sufficient to replace the population.[7] When their economic circumstances allowed them the choice, a growing proportion of young middle-class women were staying home to manage households and raise children.

Between 1952 and 1962, 316,000 registered nurses dropped out of the work force. Nursing suffered a higher proportion of inactives than did other comparable women's occupations: for nursing the inactives constituted 55 percent of the total. For secondary school teachers the inactive rate was 36 percent, for elementary school teachers 38 percent, for librarians 37 percent, and for social welfare workers 48 percent.[8] One factor was the salaries paid to nurses: at the beginning of the 1960s the pay for nursing was lower than for factory work or teaching. Nurses received little or no extra pay for overtime work, insurance and other benefits were poor, and they had little voice in their occupational governance in the work settings. Little wonder that nursing shortages were proving to be resistant to every effort toward a solution. The cards were stacked heavily against those attempting to recruit larger numbers of young people into the profession.

As a result, interest in the problems and issues of registered nursing education, including the ADN program, was widespread during the 1950s, in large part because health officials and educators continued to worry about looming nursing shortages. An article by Congresswoman Frances P. Bolton entitled "The Crisis in Health Care" appeared in April 1954. She summarized the results of her survey of 3,300 nurses, physicians, hospital administrators, government officials, and health officials, which confirmed the alarming shortage of nurses.[9] The survey also revealed the disagreements about the solutions to a problem of long standing. The respondents to her survey could not agree; health care professionals were not uniting behind any one approach to the problem. Moreover, the survey revealed the many lines of contention among nurses, physicians, hospital administrators, government officials, and others. Such lack of consensus goes a long way to explaining why Bolton's bills calling for federal aid for nursing education had run into so much trouble during the first half of the 1950s.

Representative Bolton, author of the legislation establishing the Nurse Cadet Corps program of World War II, continued after the war to work energetically in congressional circles on behalf of nursing. In 1951 she introduced a bill, H.R. 910, to establish a comprehensive federal program for nursing education. Under the program, scholarships to students as well as direct aid to schools would have been provided (in the first year, $44 million would have been directed to education for registered nurses, $3 million for practical nurses), and a new Division of Nursing Education under the direction of a nurse would have been established, advised by a National Council of Nursing Education. The program, unlike competing legislation before the House, was not a temporary measure to meet the Korean War emergency; it was to be a permanent program of the federal government.[10] The bill met with strong opposition, even before hearings began in September. Some of the opposition even came from the ranks of nurses; an ANA poll in May revealed that although 622 of 654 nursing program directors approved federal aid to nursing education in principle, 407 were opposed to anything resembling the Cadet Nurse program; 593 preferred the Bolton bill over competing legislation before Congress. The AHA national meeting of that year revealed great ambivalence toward such legislation; many administrators were wary of federal intrusion and defensive about the impact on hospital-based nursing schools. In the hearings on the bill, the AMA expressed strong opposition based on fear of the socialization of health care. Moreover, many nurses expressed strong opposition, some in the hearings, others in letters and articles in nursing journals.[11] By March of 1952 the bill was tabled, effectively dead, and Bolton warned the nation of its "gravely serious plight" in the face of the growing shortage of nurses and its inability to act decisively.[12]

In 1953, under the new Eisenhower administration, Bolton tried once more to get federal aid to nursing education enacted. Once more, the opposition was too strong. The only aid to nursing education that was winning approval in Congress at this time was that focused on aid to nursing education in psychiatric care.[13] Historians Kalisch and Kalisch have said of the congresswoman's efforts: "Mrs. Bolton had patiently and persistently used every legislative and conciliatory device at her command to advance her postwar nursing bills. She had succeeded to the degree that there was not much more room for compromise. It was now [in 1953] . . . a question of whether Congress did, in fact, want to use Federal money to stimulate nurse education."[14] Apparently, it did not; in 1955, when Bolton introduced a bill to appropriate funds simply to underwrite a study of nursing education needs, it was defeated. The AMA backed the bill but the ANA opposed it, saying its enactment would only delay concrete action.[15]

Federal Support for Faculty Preparation

Concrete action would indeed be taken, starting in the mid-1950s. The nursing shortage, among other health care issues, was simply too acute to ignore. The rapid expansion of governmental programs in nursing during the latter half of the 1950s indicates clearly how much the crisis mood propelled action at long last. The mid-1950s were watershed years for nursing education, for a new and different focus in Congress on nursing and nursing education dated from this time. Federal support for training in public health nursing had been well established ever since the Great Depression; federal support for psychiatric nurse training had been established somewhat later, in 1947. As a consequence, by the mid-1950s public health and psychiatric nursing claimed a disproportionate share of nurses trained at the postdiploma level. But now, in 1954 and 1955, pressure on the federal government to address more directly the need for stronger staff nursing in hospitals took the form of a push to establish federal programs in support of graduate training for nurses who would teach in the basic nursing education programs.

The political situation was complicated: the long-range goal of the ANA, for example, was to establish nursing education generally as a responsibility of the federal government, but strong opposition to such a high level of federal involvement in health professions education was mounted by the AMA and AHA. These were years of bitter debate over the socialization of American health care.[16] The proponents of federal funding for nursing schools had learned from their battles on behalf of ill-fated bills such as Bolton's that they had a better chance to succeed if they pressed for financial aid targeted on specific missions. The preparation of teachers for ADN and other nursing education programs was just such a cause.

The Health Amendments Act of 1956, debated through the spring and early summer, was signed into law by President Eisenhower in August.[17] This law would profoundly change the face of nursing education and directly assist ADN programs in preparing faculty. Among other provisions, it authorized the Public Health Service to establish programs to provide funds for student traineeships of several types: Title I authorized traineeships along the by now familiar lines, in public health nursing at the graduate or specialized level, but Title II broke new ground. It established traineeships for registered nurses who wished to prepare to supervise other nurses, teach in nursing programs, or administer nursing education and practice programs. In Title II, for the first time, no specialty area in nursing was designated. Students awarded the traineeships received stipends and money for tuition. Title II was funded at $2 million for the first three years, $3 million for the fourth year, and $6 million in the final year. The new program made possible the advanced training of 3,800 nurses to prepare them for teaching, administration, and supervision; ultimately, fifty-four colleges and universities took part in the program.[18]

Title II traineeships provided a needed stimulus for the preparation of faculty for ADN programs. Just how many teachers were recipients of these grants is unknown, but assistance at this time was important to the future development of the AD movement.

Massive Federal Assistance Begins

In the late summer of 1960 Lucile Petry Leone, head of the federal Division of Nursing, sent a memorandum to the surgeon general of the United States with her proposals for appointments to an advisory committee to the surgeon general on improving the nation's nursing services. This was the year that the U.S. Public Health Service reorganized its nursing divisions; the old Division of Nursing Resources and the Department of Public Health Nursing were merged, to form the Division of Nursing. The nursing advisors Leone was helping the surgeon general assemble would be known as the Surgeon General's Consultant Group on Nursing. This group would play a very important role in the positive changes in nursing and nursing education that occurred during the first half of the 1960s.[19]

The government was gearing up for a strong response not only to the nursing shortage but to the nation's health needs overall. The 1960s were the time when massive federal investments in health programs began; these were also the years when national planning for manpower needs in health care began. The early 1960s were, of course, the John F. Kennedy years, and many of the programs critical to the future of nursing were rooted in the social programs of his and, subsequently, Lyndon B. Johnson's administrations. The recommendations of the Consultant Group would not fall on deaf ears.

That group, appointed at the beginning of 1961, held its first meeting on 12 and 13 June. Chaired by Alvin C. Eurich of the Fund for the Advancement of Education, the group included nursing leaders, hospital administrators, and university officials. Among the nurses were Dean Lulu Wolf Hassenplug of UCLA School of Nursing, Marian Sheahan of NLN, and Dr. Eleanor Lambertson, head of the nursing division of Teachers College, Columbia University.[20]

The mission of the Consultant Group was to "advise him [Dr. Luther Terry, the surgeon general] on nursing needs and to identify the appropriate role of the federal government in assuring adequate nursing services for our nation."[21] At long last, the profession had an official, formal means of influencing the making of health care policy at the national level. The opportunity for nursing was unprecedented.

Because the committee members represented many different constituencies in health care and nursing, they had trouble reaching consensus on several issues. For instance, the effort to determine the proper role of the practical nurse proved to be so difficult that extra meetings became necessary. Nearly as troublesome were agreeing on the proper ratio of nurses to population, defining technical versus professional nursing, determining the extent to which the baccalaureate degree should be the primary degree in professional nursing, distinguishing the levels of nursing practice and identifying the education required for each one, and determining the type of financial assistance that would be needed to improve facilities for nursing instruction.[22]

Despite their differences, the group members shared a number of concerns. All were agreed that the nursing shortage was genuine and that it had to be solved. All believed that federal funding for nursing and nursing education needed to be increased. And there was no disagreement among them, finally, that just what the nursing role *is* needed to be determined and that standards of practice needed to be set, based on that role.[23]

The consultants found it easy to reach agreement on some of the more urgent problems facing nursing: not enough students were being recruited into nursing schools regardless of type of program, too few students were college-bound, too few nursing schools were providing an adequate education, and too few nursing schools were based in colleges and universities. Moreover, the whole system of nursing education was incoherent. The absence of a logical pattern in the overall set-up was a most serious flaw, they agreed. They recommended a study of nursing education to determine ways to work it into a coherent pattern that would more effectively prepare nurses for practice.[24]

Solutions did not lie entirely within nursing education, however. The group agreed that the social and economic status of American nurses needed to be improved if adequate numbers of new nurses were to be recruited. Moreover, the differentiation among the kinds of nurses in the work setting needed improvement. Until that could be accomplished, available personnel would continue to be used inefficiently and ineffectively.

Chairman Eurich wrote:

the nation faces a critical problem in ensuring adequate nursing services in the years ahead. The need for more nurses is urgent. . . . Lack of adequate financial resources is a basic problem. . . . In the judgment of the consultant group, if the nursing problem is to be solved, there is no alternative to federal aid. . . .

Today nursing education is at a crossroad. We need careful examination of the existing types of nursing education programs, to determine how they can be merged into a pattern that will adequately prepare the nurse to render better patient care.[25]

The Consultant Group also defined the goals for a national effort to solve the nursing problem. They estimated that the nation would need 680,000 nurses in active practice by 1970, 130,000 more than were active in the early 1960s. Achieving that level would mean a 75 percent increase in the number of nurses graduating each year.

The group finally made twenty formal recommendations: that federal funds be appropriated for stepped-up recruitment, that low-cost loans and scholarships be made available for both LPNs and RNs, that professional nurse traineeships be doubled within a five-year period, that traineeships be offered in clinical specializations, that short-term traineeships be instituted, and that a program be formed for RNs to continue at the baccalaureate level after graduating from diploma schools. The Consultant Group also recommended federal grants for the construction of prototypical education facilities, for such projects as demonstration sites for the effective use of nurses in hospital settings, for continuing education and on-the-job training projects, and for consultation and research fellowships sponsored by the Public Health Service. It also recommended that funding for research in nursing by the Public Health Service be doubled. The overall goal would be both to expand the nation's nursing schools and to improve their quality.[26]

The Consultant Group made note of the "remarkable development" in associate degree education in the field of nursing. Its report mentioned the eighty-four existing programs and predicted continuing growth.[27] But several of the sticking points about the AD movement had caused the consultant group difficulty in reaching consensus. Examples to be found in the educational system concerned the levels and kinds of nurses to be prepared, the education for each, technical versus professional practice in health care agencies, and the baccalaureate as the first professional degree.

The report of the Surgeon General's Consultant Group on Nursing was not officially released until February 1968, but its concerns and recommendations were available by 1962–1963. A preliminary report entitled *Toward Quality in Nursing: Needs and Goals* was published in 1963.[28] In it, the group asserted that the "baccalaureate program should be the minimum requirement for nurses who will assume leadership positions."[29] It also recommended that a study be made of the existing system of nursing education in the light of the responsibilities and skills needed for the highest quality of nursing care and that such a study be funded jointly by the government and by private sources.

Responding to the suggestions, ANA's Committee on Education proposed that an autonomous commission be established to design and conduct the study. It was not long before both the ANA and the NLN had appropriated funds to support a joint committee to explore the means for funding such a large task.[30] In a paper written for the joint committee, Esther Lucile Brown, author of the Brown Report of 1948, identified the two problems that she considered fundamental. The first was "the lack of delineation of the nursing role when nurses interact with members of other health groups"; the second was the slow progress in improving the nursing curriculum and increasing enrollments in baccalaureate and graduate programs. This latter point, it will be remembered, was also a concern to ADN educators, among others, for the one key to ADN development overall was the preparation of nurses to teach in these programs.[31]

Government activity to solve the health care manpower problems of the nation continued on both the executive and the legislative fronts. The Manpower Development and Training Act (Public Law 87-415) provided funding for the training of auxiliary health care workers. Under the law 15,000 persons participating in 340 projects nationwide received training in health care occupations.[32] In the meantime the Division of Nursing continued its work in studying nursing activities during a period of acute nurse shortages. Its studies in 1962 revealed that RNs were spending about one-fourth to one-third of their time on activities that could be done as well by others not trained in nursing. In fact, only about one-half of the time professional nurses worked was spent in the direct care of patients. Data on nursing care hours per patient corroborated the finding and indicated severe declines: in 1950 and 1956 patient care hours averaged 3.5; in 1959 an AHA study reported 4.69 hours, a slight rise, but by 1961 nursing care hours had plummeted to 2.5.[33]

In its deliberations and publications the Surgeon General's Consultant Group emphasized its concern that a disproportionate share of patient care was being performed by auxiliary nursing personnel. Concern among professional nurses about protecting the quality of nursing care was rising. In 1964 the NLN launched its program for accrediting the nation's schools for practical nurses.

General concern was growing at that time that the education of the practical nurse was monitored too little. The NLNE Committee on the Function of Nursing in 1950 knew of only 58 practical nursing schools in the nation that were approved, but it surmised that 300 or more were in existence and lacking approval. The ANA's 1949 edition of *Facts About Nursing* stated that as of 1 January 1949 there were 2,579 students enrolled in 71 schools of practical nursing approved by state boards of nurse examiners. In any event, it was clear that many more practical nurses were practicing than were being graduated from approved schools and that their educational preparation was open to question. Whether the schools should be upgraded to ADN programs was a question that would loom large in the future.

At the beginning of 1963 President John F. Kennedy sent to Congress a major statement about his administration's policy on health. His program addressed five areas besides mental health and retardation, which he had previously supported: (1) the shortage of health care personnel, (2) the need for new health facilities, (3) the need for better care for the aged, (4) the importance of protecting citizens from pollutants in the air, in water, in drugs, and in cosmetics, and (5) the need to protect the health of the nation's children. He stressed the health manpower problem: "the harsh fact of the matter is that we are already hard hit by a critical shortage in our supply of professional health personnel, with the situation threatening to become even more critical in the years ahead."[34]

Kennedy also asked for an amendment to the Hill-Burton Act that would underwrite the cost of modernizing or replacing existing health care facilities and provide $50 million in new funds for nursing home construction. He called for legislation that would provide financial assistance to nursing students and support for graduate programs in nursing. The purpose of the latter request was twofold: to increase the number of qualified nursing teachers and to encourage more research dedicated to finding better ways to use the nurses that were available. The Kennedy program did not focus wholly on nursing, of course; he also asked for insurance and loan programs for group medical practices, the expansion of health care programs for immigrant workers, and funding for research projects in international health and medicine.[35]

On 24 September 1963 Kennedy signed into law the Health Professions Education Assistance Act (Public Law 88-129), which provided construction grants for medical, nursing, and other professional schools. It also provided scholarships and loans for students in medicine, dentistry, and osteopathy. It was funded for three years at $175 million.[36]

In January of 1964 the U.S. Public Health Service and the NLN surveyed 848 hospitals and 104 junior colleges, asking what their present enrollment capacities were and what plans they might have for construction. In all, 760 hospitals and 92 junior colleges responded; their answers made it painfully clear that the facilities needed to meet the demand were lacking. The Consultant Group had projected a goal of 680,000 nurses by 1970, which represented a 69 percent increase, but existing nursing school capacities would permit only a 31 percent increase.[37]

By mid-February of 1964 the government had received from nursing schools around the country forty-three letters of intent to build. By October, the first six construction grants had been awarded to schools of nursing.[38]

Federal Nursing Legislation Comes of Age: The Nurse Training Act of 1964

As important as the construction funds were to the future of nursing education, other legislation on the congressional agenda would be even more critical to the profession. In January 1964 Lucile Petry Leone, now the chief nurse officer of the Public Health Service, notified the ANA-NLN Coordinating Council of upcoming legislation in President Johnson's health program that included measures of importance to nursing. Johnson formally submitted his program to Congress on 10 February. He described it as the most significant nursing legislation in the nation's history.[39]

Wilbur Cohen, at the time the assistant secretary for legislation in the Department of Health, Education, and Welfare, explained the timing of this new legislation, which was focused so exclusively on nursing. He pointed out that "once you had the 1963 act" the next steps were "easy": "Once you break the back of the ideological opposition, then all you are arguing about is money. . . . You had to start with physicians and dentists, because they are the elite, they had the political power." Once these groups were being funded, the passage of nursing legislation was "relatively easy."[40]

The Nurse Training Act would authorize the appropriation of $283 million for five years. Funds could be used to finance construction for associate degree, baccalaureate, and higher degree programs, as well as for diploma programs. The funds could also be used to rehabilitate or replace existing facilities, to underwrite grants to improve the quality of teaching, to fund traineeships in professional nursing (the Nurse Traineeship Program then in existence was due to expire in June 1964), and to finance student loans. The act would also establish a national advisory council on nurse training.[41]

Hearings on the bill were held before the House Committee on Interstate and Foreign Commerce, Subcommittee on Public Health and Safety during April. Representatives of the ANA, the NLN, and several nursing schools testified in favor of the bill.[42] The act ultimately won congressional approval, and the president signed it into law on 1 September 1964. The Nurse Training Act of 1964 proved to be just as Johnson had described it, the landmark legislation for nursing in American history.

The administration's goal in backing the legislation was to increase the supply of nurses in the United States by as many as 130,000 by 1970, but the impact of the act would be far more than numerical. It provided $90 million for construction to begin in 1966, $35 million for four years of financial assistance to collegiate schools of nursing, $55 million for construction of associate degree and diploma facilities, $17 million in special project grants, $50 million for the continuation of nurse traineeships for five more years, $41 million in formula grants for diploma programs ($100 per year per student), and $85 million for student loans in all accredited nursing programs regardless of type. (Loans were 90 percent financed by the government, 10 percent by the schools.) The loan program was intended to attract as many new people into nursing as possible: students could borrow up to $1,000 a year, they could repay over ten years beginning one year after graduation, and the loan would be forgiven at prorated percentages depending on the number of years the borrower remained active in nursing service.[43] The ADN programs were to reap the benefits.

Responding to recommendations and pressure from the American Hospital Association, the Senate added to the program $17 million in special project grants for hospital-based diploma programs.[44] With support for collegiate nursing education in the ascendancy, the supporters of hospital programs were clearly engaging in rearguard action. The bulk of federal support would be directed to nursing programs based in junior colleges and universities.

Implementation of the act began immediately after its enactment, and proceeded quickly. To be eligible for funds, a school, if it were not already accredited, had to be reasonably sure of accreditation by the NLN. Before the end of 1964 the league had developed its criteria for such "reasonable assurance" for purposes of the act. The national advisory council established under the act, whose purpose was to advise as to policies and procedures and to review schools' applications for funds, first met on 1 and 2 February 1965.[45]

The first task facing federal officials was the huge job of explaining the act to the nation's nursing educators. Between October 1964 and March 1965 the NLN and state nurses' associations sponsored meetings in forty-six states to do just that. At these meetings representatives of the Division of Nursing reached a grand total of 6,000 persons. In addition, fact sheets were sent to all schools of nursing.[46]

It was soon clear that the word had been spread effectively and that the needs of nursing education were indeed great. The traineeship program appropriation of $8 million was easily exhausted during the first year. Grants for special projects, to be awarded according to criteria developed by the National Advisory Council, were much sought after by ADN educators. The grant review panel of eight nursing education experts met in late May 1965 to recommend the funding of thirty-nine projects in twenty-one states, the District of Columbia, and Puerto Rico. The staff responsible for awarding construction grants made thirty-five site visits and consulted with the NLN to determine space requirements for nursing education facilities. This work culminated in the publication of a guide for planners entitled *Nursing Education Facilities, Programing Considerations and Architectural Guide*, which reports the committee's advice to the Public Health Service concerning policies for funding the construction of new schools and the expansion of existing ones.[47]

A fund totaling more than $3 million was established for student loans in 402 schools for the fiscal year 1965. By 1966 the number of schools had risen to 558, and the only states not participating in the loan program were Delaware and Alaska. The number of students borrowing funds by the end of the first year of the program's operation reached 3,645, or 5 percent of the total nursing school enrollment in the nation.[48]

Clearly, the federal impact on nursing and nursing education during the late 1960s would be great. Associate degree nursing education would benefit. The growth of the ADN idea up to this point had been vigorous, but with the infusion of federal funds across so broad a front—including construction grants and student loans—the new programs would continue their rapid growth. In 1964 the ADN programs in the United States represented but 11 percent of all RN programs; just three years later, in 1967, their proportion had exactly doubled, to 22 percent.[49]

The Nurse Training Act's accreditation requirements plus the rapid increase in the number of ADN programs necessitated structural changes in the NLN. Until a by-laws change creating a separate ADN council or department could be approved by the entire membership, the league established a separate Associate Degree Program Unit. Gerald J. Griffin became its first director in August 1965. During this same period, interest in the joint NLN-AAJC Committee on Nursing Education was reawakened, and national conferences on ADN education were being planned.[50]

The National Focus on Health Care

An idea that gained widespread acceptance during the 1960s was that all citizens have a right to good health care. Certainly, much of the nation's attention was focused on health and health care issues. The Nurse Training Act was but one facet of the national preoccupation.

In 1966 President Johnson appointed the National Advisory Commission on Health Manpower to recommend action by government or by private institutions, organizations, or individuals for improving the availability and use of health manpower. The commission concluded that there was a crisis in American health care.

The crisis, however, is not simply one of numbers. It is true that substantially increased numbers of health manpower will be needed over time. But if additional personnel are employed in the present manner and within the present patterns and systems of care, they will not avert, or even perhaps alleviate, the crisis. *Unless we improve the system* through which health care is provided, care will continue to become less satisfactory, even though there are massive increases in cost and in numbers of health personnel.[51]

The commission released its report in November of 1967. In emphasizing the lack of a coherent health care system in the United States, it noted that increases in health care costs were twice the size of increases in other areas and that public dissatisfaction was also rising. It predicted that by 1975 the health care sector would be the nation's leading employer and asserted the commissioners' belief that all health care education should be conducted by colleges and universities.[52]

The Division of Nursing, seeking to grasp more clearly the nursing manpower situation, in 1966 contracted with Stewart Altman, an economist, to do a study of nursing shortages and projections for the future.

Also in 1966 the Comprehensive Health Planning Act was signed into law. Its preamble stated that the fulfillment of the national purposes depended on our "promoting and assuring the highest level of health attainable for every person." The Partnership for Health Program, instituted in 1966, provided federal support for areawide health planning. The belief that the system itself stood in need of reform was clearly becoming a widely accepted notion, as increasingly the federal government's programs in health reflected this concern for the ways that the overall system might be made to work more effectively.

A concomitant development was highlighted by the nation's surgeon general, William Stewart. He pointed out that the scientific revolution had accelerated specialization among physicians, which in turn had forced specialization in nursing, requiring professional nurses to take on new and complex responsibilities.[53] This process, together with the trend toward comprehensive health planning and the determination to solve health manpower problems, would make its mark on ADN education over the next decade. All these various concerns would affect the way people perceived two issues concerning the two-year nursing degree, its place among other nursing programs, and its role in the health care system as a whole. There would be little agreement on either issue.

Contemporary Assessments of the Nurse Training Act

Under the provisions of the Nurse Training Act much money and effort were poured into nursing education during the first three years after its enactment. By 1967, fully 18 percent of all students enrolled in nursing —17,218—were borrowing money. The average loan was for $567, which was about the same as the average loan to students at the time under the National Defense Student Loan Program. (By 1968 the proportion of student nurses borrowing funds had risen to 23 percent.) In addition, 248 schools awarded Educational Opportunity grants averaging $325 to about 7,000 students. An average of $8,000 was paid to 447 diploma schools of nursing. Project grants totaling $14.5 million had been awarded to 108 sponsoring nursing schools. The $47 million in federal funds devoted to the Traineeship Program had made possible 8,000 traineeships and 18,000 short-term courses.

A committee appointed by the secretary of the Department of Health, Education, and Welfare completed an official review of the first three years of the Nurse Training Act at the end of 1967, after having met in May, July, September, and October.[54] In its report the committee noted the shortage of leaders in nursing, especially teachers, and was particularly alarmed at the continuing use of auxiliary personnel at high rates. It made nine recommendations:

1. That the Nurse Training Act be extended for five more years.
2. That the federal share for construction grants be increased to 75 percent, that loans be made available to help schools meet the matching requirements, and that funds be used to build continuing education facilities.
3. That basic support grants be extended to all types of nursing education programs and that basic start-up grants be available to universities not having medical centers.
4. That grants be extended to hospitals and other agencies for projects to improve nursing education, to help schools achieve accreditation, and to update the skills of inactive nurses.
5. That training grants under the Professional Nurse Traineeship Program be increased to include administrative costs, scholarships, and loans up to $2,500 a year.
6. That funds be used for recruitment, state and regional planning, and identifying nursing talent among the disadvantaged.
7. That funds for nursing research be increased.

8. That staffing and funds for travel costs for consultation be increased.
9. That support for the Division of Nursing be increased, to make it stronger.[55]

From 1964, when the Nurse Training Act was enacted, to 1967, when its impact was being so closely scrutinized, the nursing shortage had grown even more acute. By some estimates, 150,000 additional nurses were needed. At the same time, 300,000 RNs were licensed but not working. Existing hospital beds were being closed as a result of the shortage, and many worried about the serious repercussions of the poor care that resulted. Both the U.S. Public Health Service and the American Hospital Association concluded that 80,000 more RNs and 40,000 more LPNs were needed immediately. In addition, 50,000 aides were needed in general hospitals, and 30,000 in mental hospitals.[56]

Adding to the burden was the drain on health care manpower caused by the escalation of hostilities in Vietnam during this period. The Army Nurse Corps needed 1,800 more RNs to reach its authorized strength of 5,000. The Air Corps awarded the warrant officer status to AD nurses in an attempt to reach its full strength, as it needed more air evacuation nurses.[57]

Then on 17 August the president signed the Health Manpower Act of 1968 into law. This was an omnibus bill amending five separate laws, including the Nurse Training Act of 1964. Under the amendment the act was extended another four years, and the NLN lost its status as the sole accrediting institution for nursing education programs.[58] The appropriation for nurse training for 1970 was $115 million, and $145 million was the projected total for 1971. The amended act strengthened the scholarship program; traineeships were continued, and the expenditures for construction grants were expected to total between $15 and $19 million. Institutional formula grants had been proposed but were not funded.[59]

The nursing shortage continued unabated. Turnover rates in hospitals were high: one study by the Division of Nursing found that the turnover rate among nurses was 50 percent. The rates would climb higher even than that in coming years. The attrition was such that in 1968 manpower specialists were declaring, "we have to graduate 20,000 more nurses a year just to keep up."[60] (Graduations that year from professional nursing schools totaled just over 41,000.[61])

In 1968 about half of the nation's people in health care occupations were nurses. There were more than a million RNs, but fewer than half of them were employed full-time as nurses, and another 150,000 worked in nursing half-time. In addition, there were 320,000 LPNs and 800,000 aides, orderlies, and attendants. It was expected that federally funded refresher courses could bring as many as 10,000 RNs back into the field, but it was clear that the shortages needed to be more clearly defined as to levels and kinds of practice needed by the health care system. Even as that system expanded, its needs kept changing, making the planning problem more difficult.[62]

The federal government released $1 million in priority funding to underwrite refresher courses that it was hoped would bring 3,500 nurses back to work in the near future. Federal officials also turned their attention to the recruitment of disadvantaged students. For example, the California State College Foundation received a federal grant to recruit Mexican-American students, and career mobility programs for practical nurses were instituted in 1969. In another instance, the Division of Nursing sponsored a project at Hunter College of the City University of New York to educate LPNs for RN licensure—a seventeen-month work-study program based in New York City public hospitals.[63]

The increasingly common ADN programs figured more and more prominently in all such efforts by the federal government, for they were often the schools most accessible, both geographically and economically, to the target populations. In a word, as the nursing shortage intensified and public determination to overcome the problem and extend health care equally also rose, a secure future in nursing education for the ADN program became more and more certain.

As planning for the expansion of nursing education facilities grew more complex and as planning became more and more a process mandated under the law, the collection of facts about nursing practice and education improved visibly. In 1969 the Division of Nursing arranged with the Bureau of the Census for a survey of the condition of nursing school facilities in 1,270 state-approved schools of nursing. Until the late 1960s, any such surveys of the field had been left to nursing itself, whose professional associations were poorly equipped and inadequately funded to undertake scientific national studies. The 1969 survey was a first. It assessed each facility for the ages, sizes, types, and conditions of the buildings, even their accessibility and the suitability of their locations.[64]

Federal appropriations for nursing under the Nurse Training Act continued at a high level: traineeships were slated to receive nearly $10.5 million; scholarships $6.5 million; construction grants $8 million, $3.2 million of which was allotted for associate degree and diploma programs; and projects $4 million. The only cuts in the support were for construction and research projects; other budget items represented increased expenditures.[65]

As the ADN program began to establish itself as the program most likely to grow rapidly and the federal government became more directly involved in the planning and financing of nursing education and of individual programs, the nursing profession entered a painful period of internal change. The full impact of the ADN on nursing and nursing education is not comprehensible until one takes a close look at the profession's internal struggles during the first half of the 1960s. That story is the subject of the next chapter.

Upheaval Within:

The Politics of the Profession

The growth of ADN education during the 1950s was steady, but it was nothing next to the explosion of the 1960s, when at times a new ADN program was opening somewhere in the country every week. One reason for the rapid expansion was federal financial assistance to nursing education; another was the rising concern among Americans over health and social issues, especially those regarding equal access to health care and to educational opportunity for all citizens.

Even as ADN education grew explosively, the nursing shortage continued unabated. Public preoccupation with health issues grew, in response not only to manpower shortages but also to the greatly increased specialization of health care practice and the greater demands this placed on the health professions and facilities. The national nursing organizations struggled to deal with the largely unforeseen consequences of the increasing controversy about nursing education and to sort out their respective roles among themselves. Not only health care but the nation itself was passing through a time of upheaval. The civil rights and women's movements arose, confrontational politics exploded into violence at times, the Vietnam War grew into a deeply divisive issue, and the very social fabric at times seemed to be at risk. Few, if any, of these issues proved to be irrelevant to nursing. The strain of dealing with them took its toll on the profession.

In the late spring of 1950 the six existing national nursing organizations endorsed a plan for reorganizing themselves into two units. They would form the American Nurses' Association, for nurses alone, and the National League of America, which included others besides nurses as members. The latter was subsequently renamed the National League for Nursing. The league would incorporate into its structure the Committee for the Improvement of Nursing Services.[1] The reorganization was completed by 1952. The task of fostering the development and promoting excellence in nursing education fell to the NLN.

During the mid-1950s NLN effort to promote the educational arm was quite active. It provided an increasing number of workshops and conferences of interest to its educational constituents. In 1958, for example, it held eleven conferences on nursing curricula, and six of its subcommittees met to discuss the NLN's position on the future of nursing education.[2] This same year, members of the ANA adopted a resolution at their national convention in which they assumed the responsibility for the improvement of standards of nursing competence; it was assumed that such standards could not be divorced from concern about the standards of education. The ANA Committee on Current and Long-Term Goals urged the delegates to promote "educational standards of professional calibre," and the improvement of all standards became one of the three priorities of the national organization.[3]

Within a year the ANA leadership had assumed the position that the education of all RNs should be located in institutions of higher education. Their stand was based on the belief that the hospital system of nursing education was inadequate, a conclusion that had been reached repeatedly by nursing leaders during the twentieth century. The sentiments were hardly new, of course, but what was new was the fact that the profession's national association was making the stand official, designating it as a program priority. The profession would now push much more concertedly to move nursing education out of the hospital and onto the nation's campuses. That campaign would only add impetus to the ADN movement.

Moving ahead with an educational agenda, in April of 1960 the ANA's Committee on Current and Long-Term Goals recommended to the national association's board of directors that the following goal be presented to the 1960 House of Delegates for approval and action:

> To insure that within the next 20–30 years, the education basic to the professional practice of nursing, for those who enter the profession, shall be secured in a program that provides the intellectual, technical and cultural components of both a professional and liberal education. Toward this end, the ANA shall promote the baccalaureate program ultimately so that in due course it becomes the basic educational foundation for professional nursing.[4]

Goal 3, as it was called, was a shot taken directly across the bows of both ADN and diploma education, or so it seemed to their proponents. Many graduates of ADN and diploma programs believed that they were entering professional practice and that this goal, were it realized, would exclude them from first-class status. With the issuance of Goal 3, the ANA goals committee brought to a boil issues that had long been simmering: *Could* the educational system of the nation and *would* the profession accept the baccalaureate degree as minimal preparation for professional practice?

In 1960 all three types of nursing schools were preparing nurses for practice that many considered professional. The outsider might well —and often did—ask why, if the graduates of all three were equally qualified as RNs, there were three programs at all, and not just one. Or, alternatively, if the programs were distinctly different and producing different graduates, why were the distinctions ignored, that is, why were these graduates lumped together in the workplace into one group? Why did all of them take the same licensing examination?

A nurse is a nurse is a nurse, quipped many in response. Others disagreed, often vociferously. As the Consultant Group in the federal government noted, the educational structure in nursing was illogical. Not only that, it did not fit the way the profession was structured in the real world of employment and practice.[5]

Resolving the controversy, everyone knew, would not be easy. In point of fact, many issues were involved, not just one. The oldest issue was the quarrel over hospital-based versus collegiate education for nursing, joined, as we have seen in earlier chapters, by the hospital schools and the earliest baccalaureate programs in nursing. The ADN programs logically belonged to the collegiate side. But another issue was implicit in the ANA committee's Goal 3, which set the four-year baccalaureate program at a level above the two shorter programs, the diploma and the ADN. The newcomer, the technical nurse movement, thus found itself in the swing position, situated on one or the other side of the dividing line, depending on where the line was drawn.

Yet another issue concerned the vested interests that were involved. Any change in the present system would mean that someone's program was in danger. Leaders in diploma and associate degree nursing education feared to lose whatever advantages they held. Few directors of existing programs relished the idea that their kind of program might have to close or accept reduced status or lose hegemony to the others.

Although most people in nursing at the beginning of the 1960s agreed that the existing situation was unacceptable and that the illogicalities cried out for solution, there was little consensus as to what would be best for the profession or for the public it served. For this reason, the ANA board of directors chose in 1960 to present the recommendation of the goals committee to the House of Delegates not for a vote but instead for information and study during the 1960–1962 biennium (the ANA delegates met every other year, not annually). And in May 1960 the House of Delegates accepted the recommendation as a basis for continued discussion at the state level in addition to the plank that stated their intention to continue to elevate the educational requirements of nursing education by formulating standards essential to effective nursing practice.

Thus was launched a series of events that would lead to a period of great upheaval among nurses, much of it focused on the stands regarding the future of nursing education taken by the two leading nursing associations: the ANA's 1965 "Position Paper" and the NLN's "Resolution 5" of the same year. (So widely were they debated that formal titles were virtually forgotten; to this day, reference to the ANA's stand is made simply with the phrase "the Position Paper." Resolution 5, also supporting the movement of nursing education into colleges and universities, is presented in detail below.)

This first step, taken by the ANA, provoked controversy over the proper respective roles of the ANA and the NLN. In June of 1961 the ANA board of directors propelled further the association's drift into the province of nursing education when it approved the creation of the Committee on Education. Until now, the two leading nursing organizations, the ANA and the NLN, had operated with little difficulty on the understanding that their purposes and focuses were different. Heretofore, nursing education had clearly been the NLN's central mission. In response to the ANA move, the NLN worried that the ANA was "getting into an area which rightfully belonged to the League."[6] The issue was important enough to leaders of both organizations that they formed study committees that met in June and September 1961 to discuss their respective responsibilities.

The NLN's own position had been defined earlier by its Study Committee on Goals and Purposes, appointed by the NLN board of directors. It was asked to provide the criteria that "will enable us to judge whether . . . some of these principles listed under ANA are appropriate for ANA, NLN, or both."[7] Mary Louise Brown, chair, presented the following criteria for those activities for which more than one nursing organization might share responsibility: "(1) responsibility [for an activity] is shared by more than one segment of the [nursing] community; (2) planning and programming are accomplished by the concerted action of participants from more than one segment of the community; and (3) performance requires human and financial resources in excess of those than can be supplied by any one occupational group."[8]

The ANA's position was stated in its "Report of the Study Committee on the Functions of ANA," adopted by the House of Delegates in May of 1962. When the NLN bylaws were adopted in 1952, it said, there were assigned to the NLN "functions which no other professional organization had formally assigned to a voluntary organization concerned with providing its service to the community." Further, "no provisions were made in the by-laws of the new organization for NLN to accept from ANA statements of standards and goals to guide that organization in its efforts to improve nursing education and service to the community." The report emphasized the ANA's belief that the two organizations would be complementary and that the NLN would accord the ANA the traditional prerogatives of a professional association. The ANA pointed out that, given the fact that the NLN's membership included others besides nurses—agencies and professional educators not having nursing degrees, for example—it might be that "all of the functions allocated to NLN are not appropriate to such an organization—that some should be assumed by the professional association."[9] The ANA was moving aggressively to assume responsibility for making decisions in the arena of nursing education.

In short, then, the ANA's work on Goal 3 exposed yet another of the lines that divided the nursing profession into separate camps. The problem was not simply how to manage the relations between the profession's two leading organizations. The question at the heart of the matter was this: Who would have the right to speak for all of nursing on this most delicate of issues raised in Goal 3? Which organization—the one generally focused on nursing education and including among its members people who were not professional nurses or the one made up exclusively of nurses and speaking for the profession as a profession—should define the education required for practice?

As the two organizations wrestled with the problem of their respective roles, they continued to consider the issues expressed in the ANA's

Goal 3, that is, the consequences of designating the baccalaureate degree as the minimum requirement for entry into professional nursing practice. In January of 1960 (four months before the ANA committee voted on its Goal 3) the NLN board of directors had decided to appoint a new committee, the Committee on Perspectives, to consider "the future of the nursing profession . . . and to call to the attention of the Board issues or questions of import in planning for the future." The new committee was a direct descendant of the Committee on the Future, whose findings and recommendations had been published in *Nurses for a Growing Nation*.[10] John Millis, president of Western Reserve University and a member of the NLN board, suggested "a group of individuals interested, dedicated, and knowledgeable . . . who are sufficiently in touch with the basic forces in our society and specifically with[in] the [nursing] profession . . . to be able to forecast some of the long term trends." He envisioned a group able to "flow from one problem to another . . . one area of service to another; now education, now service—at a practical and professional nurse level"—a group, in short, of breadth of vision, not wearing parochial blinders.[11]

The committee members who were appointed included such prominent nurses as Margaret Ainstein, Sister Charles Marie, Marian Sheahan, Ruth Freeman (who served as chair), Mary Kelly Mullane, and Ella Allison; a physician, Sidney M. Greenberg, associate professor of clinical medicine, New York Hospital-Cornell Medical Center; and others prominent in the consideration of health care issues: John Millis, Mary C. Rockefeller, and Robert Strauss, chairman of the Department of Behavioral Science of the University of Kentucky Medical Center.[12]

The committee met several times over a three-year period and explored three subjects: the nature of the patient and the current composition of the patient census, the mix of personnel involved in patient care, and the agencies providing the care and the education of the people providing the services.[13] The committee quickly recognized that the answers to many of the problems confronting nursing lay within the province of nursing education, but despite that, it made no attempt to suggest ways to reshape the system of nursing education. The committee saw its role as being, not the judge of the changes in nursing education that were being recommended, but of "sounding the alert to the factors that are impeding some of these changes." In so defining its role, the committee concentrated on the exploration of what nurses would need to know in twenty years, not on weighing the relative worth of the various nursing education programs.[14] In short, the committee would take no stand on Goal 3 or Resolution 5.

The NLN, however, did have an official position regarding nursing that it wished to define and disseminate. Early in 1961 that statement was completed and was published under the title "Opportunities for Education in Nursing."[15] The position spelled out in this publication, adopted by the NLN delegates in convention, supported all four types of nursing education programs—baccalaureate, diploma, associate degree, and practical nursing. The statement said virtually nothing about the future but instead explained and supported the existing educational structure for nursing. The NLN, for the moment, would take a conservative tack.[16]

In 1962 the ANA board of directors appointed the members to the previously approved Committee on Education, with the following charges: first, to recommend ways the association could meet its specific responsibilities in nursing education; second, to formulate the basic principles of education that are essential for effective nursing practice; and third, to study the effect of federal and state legislation on nursing education and formulate recommendations based on the findings.

The NLN in 1964 began to redirect its attention more to the future of nursing education. In October the Steering Committee of the NLN's Division of Nursing Education appointed the Committee on Nursing Education, which was to undertake the following task: "to look at the future of nursing education in consideration of the NLN Committee on Perspectives report and Resolution #5; define the steps that need to be taken; study the concept of change and its effect on educational programs; and chart a course for the future of NLN in nursing education."[17]

The resolution referred to was the NLN's first definitive stand on the future of nursing education. It was based largely on the publication entitled *Perspectives for Nursing*.[18] With this resolution, the NLN took a position that was sympathetic toward higher education for nurses but nonetheless expressed the belief that hospital schools of nursing would continue to carry the major part of the load for some time to come. (In 1965 diploma schools indeed comprised 69 percent of all programs for professional nurses.[19]) However, the league took care to hedge: "This does not rule out the eventual shift that will place nurse education wholly within higher education institutions."[20]

But the league was not alone in choosing to move with caution. In

January 1964 the ANA board of directors agreed that action on its Goal 3 should not be taken at the June convention. The Committee on Education urged the board to postpone action until a "scrupulous examination of the following issues and concerns" could be taken: "the differentiation of practice at the professional and technical levels, an analysis of Goal 3 and its ramifications, consideration of trends in general and professional education, and consideration of current and predicted changes within the culture."[21] In June the ANA House of Delegates did adopt a motion that "ANA continue to work toward baccalaureate education as the educational foundation for professional nursing practice." Delegates requested that the Committee on Education work with "all deliberate speed to enunciate a precise definition of preparation for nursing at all levels."[22] This was the request that culminated in the association's issuance in 1965 of the hotly debated Position Paper.

1965: Year of Crisis and Dissent

The year 1965 was a watershed year for Americans generally, as the nation formally entered the conflict in Vietnam and its youth expressed ever more vociferously its disagreement with the government's policies. Nursing, too, engaged in debate over its future directions at a new, more intense level.

On 24 September 1965 the ANA board of directors endorsed *A Position Paper on Educational Preparation for Nurse Practitioners and Assistants to Nurses*, known ever after simply as "the Position Paper."[23] This was the ANA's first definitive statement on nursing education. The main assumption guiding the development of the paper was that "education for those in the health professions must increase (in depth and breadth) as scientific knowledge expands." According to the members of the Committee on Education, the purpose of the paper was to describe a system of education, not to attach labels to practitioners.[24] The position set forth can be summarized briefly.

First, it was asserted that the education for all those who are licensed to practice nursing should take place in institutions of higher education. This was nothing more than a restatement of the fundamental recommendation of the Brown Report, issued seventeen years earlier.

Second, it was asserted that the minimum preparation for beginning professional practice *at the present time*, not at some future date, should be the baccalaureate degree in nursing. The refusal to put this off as a goal for realization in the future was the most controversial feature of this white paper.

Third, the paper described the associate degree in nursing as being currently the minimum preparation for beginning technical nursing practice. The word *technical* of course echoed Mildred Montag's own terminology at the outset of the ADN experiment, but its definition by this time had become a subject of heated debate.

Fourth, the paper declared that education for assistants in health care occupations should be short, intensive pre-service programs in vocational education institutions, not on-the-job training programs.

The ANA also asserted its intention to continue supporting all three categories of nurses delivering health care services: the professional, the technical, and the assistive.

During the 1966 ANA convention the House of Delegates commended the board of directors and the Committee on Education for "their farsighted action" in issuing the position paper on education and adopted it as the official position of the association.[25] To add fuel to the fire, the ANA Committee on Membership proposed that the board of directors adopt a new position: beginning with the membership year 1975, it was proposed, a baccalaureate degree in nursing from a school accredited by the NLN would be a requirement for new members then and thereafter entering the ANA.[26] The negative response was so strong that the position was reversed by the following January.

In December of 1965 the ANA also published the text of the Position Paper in its official journal, the *American Journal of Nursing*. The implications of the structure it recommended were spelled out: "Some diploma schools would begin to participate in programs with colleges or universities in the development of baccalaureate programs; others would participate with junior colleges in planning the development of junior college programs." It was expected that diploma hospital-based programs would begin to close, and the hope was expressed that practical nurse programs would be replaced with programs for "beginning technical practice in junior and community colleges."[27] (Note that it was just the preceding year that the NLN had begun its program for accrediting LPN programs.)

At this time, at the end of 1965, approximately 78 percent of all nurses in practice were graduates of hospital-based diploma programs, a very large portion of the whole profession. Concern was of course expressed immediately about the impact on these nurses of the restructuring recommended in the Position Paper. In response, the ANA board of directors spent the next months preparing a publication that they issued in September 1966. *A Date with the Future*, a brochure, interpreted the meaning of the Position Paper for graduates of hospital schools of nursing. The brochure was meant to reassure the diploma graduate that her own position was not jeopardized by the Position Paper.[28]

During the same months when the ANA was setting off the controversy over its Position Paper, the NLN was also defining its stand in regard to nursing education: its Resolution 5 was adopted in May 1965. It, too, expressed support for the movement of nursing education toward institutions of higher education, but it took a more cautious route than the ANA, expressing the belief that the hospital programs would carry the load in nursing education for some time to come. Essentially, Resolution 5, adopted in convention at San Francisco, supported

1. the trend toward college-based programs;
2. community planning for the orderly movement of nursing education into institutions of higher learning;
3. immediate expedition of recruiting efforts;
4. a vigorous campaign to interpret the different kinds of initial preparation for personnel prepared to perform complementary but different functions.

The NLN board of directors called the times a period of "inevitable change in nursing education" and seemed to believe that a wait-and-see posture was the wisest course.[29]

The years 1965 to 1968 saw an overwhelmingly negative response to both the ANA Position Paper and Resolution 5. Contributing to the reaction was the fact that as of 1966 nearly 86 percent of all employed RNs were hospital-school graduates who had not progressed beyond that level of education. The proportion of hospital-based programs among all basic nursing programs was down slightly, from 69 percent to 65 percent, but they still accounted for 65 percent of all nursing students enrolled and graduated 71 percent of all novices.[30]

Nevertheless, the paper did garner some support: nurse educators by and large defended it, and the Conference of Catholic Schools of Nursing backed it. That almost all its defenders during this period were educators only emphasized yet another line of division in the profession: that marking the separation of the practitioners from the academicians. Their battle, an old one for other professional groups, was heating up.

Nurses could define themselves as belonging to one of two cultures —the one centering on academic and clinical aspirations or the one centering on actual practice.

As debate continued, the ANA continued to issue interpretive statements to clarify the meaning of the Position Paper. In the meantime, the NLN was contending with the increasingly adverse reaction to its Resolution 5. Nursing education had become the divisive problem of nursing, the issue that was debated at every turn and that dominated the pages of nursing journals and newsletters.

In June of 1966 the ANA board of directors continued to move aggressively in education by adopting a motion that "appropriate groups within ANA be encouraged to develop standards" on the qualifications, use, distribution, and numbers of nurses needed to provide care in the health care system.[31]

In January 1967 the NLN Committee on Nursing Education, appointed to study and clarify Resolution 5, responded by developing its own Statement on Nursing Education, which was subsequently adopted by the NLN board. The statement strongly reaffirmed Resolution 5. It described several developments of profound importance to nursing that had arisen since the resolution was first framed. These included the shortage of faculty in all types of nursing programs, the imbalance in ratios of different types of nursing personnel in health care agencies, the unprecedented growth of nursing programs in junior and senior colleges and universities, the rapid closing of hospital-based diploma programs, and the trend toward care of patients by unprepared and unsupervised nurses. The statement urged community planning for change, urging especially the expansion of associate degree and baccalaureate programs.[32] The statement concluded with the assertion that until the goals of Resolution 5 could be realized, the NLN had the obligation to assist all types of nursing programs, from practical nursing to master's-level programs.[33]

The Reaction of Hospital-Based Programs

Opponents of the resolution worked hard to have the league rescind Resolution 5; their hope was that this could be accomplished at the May 1967 national convention of the NLN. The Resolutions Committee, however, strongly recommended support for the resolution because it "does not represent a departure but rather an evolving process." Board

members were persuaded that the opposition was based on a misinter-
pretation of the league's position regarding hospital-based programs. That
position, the board agreed, had been defined in a joint statement the
NLN made with the American Hospital Association in February 1967,
which concluded with these words: "We issue this statement to demonstrate an active and joint support at this time of all accredited programs, including those in hospital schools, in their efforts to improve
nursing care of the American people through the production of qualified
nursing personnel."[34]

At a meeting held before the convention, on May 5, the board discussed a letter to league president Lois Austin from Ruth Sleeper, chairman of the NLN Department of Diploma Programs steering committee; Sleeper's letter expressed the concerns of the Council of Member
Agencies, voiced in its most recent meeting. The letter was sent at the
direction of the majority of the 1,104 representatives of 555 agencies,
with the request that it be read at both the board meeting and the business meeting of the NLN in convention. The council's concerns were
as follows:

1. Diploma programs lacked representation on the ANA-NLN Committee on Nursing Careers.
2. They were not proportionately represented on the committee that
   prepared the statement on nursing education.
3. Only a small number of diploma school representatives appeared on
   the ballot for national offices in NLN.
4. No diploma school representatives had been appointed members of
   the NLN nominating committee.
5. Continued use of the word *technical* to describe diploma program
   graduates was incorrect and misleading.
6. Priority was being given by NLN to the recruitment of students for
   associate degree and baccalaureate programs.

Miss Sleeper's letter added that "the feelings of the representatives were
so intense that a suggestion was made to withdraw financial support
from NLN and create a new and separate organization for diploma
schools."[35]

All efforts to have the NLN rescind Resolution 5 failed. But as a result
of the challenge by the Council on Diploma Programs, in January 1969
the NLN board withdrew the 1967 Statement on Nursing Education in
the belief that it did not reflect after all the entire league's position.[36]

In 1968 the American Hospital Association offered institutional membership in AHA to hospital-based diploma programs. By September of that year 230 schools had joined and in November the Assembly of Hospital Schools held its second meeting. The divisions in nursing were becoming increasingly sharp, and the rifts between the separate educational camps were visibly wider. Many nursing leaders began to worry that the divisiveness would do the profession great harm.

In January 1970 the ANA Commission on Nursing Education reported its progress on a working paper dealing with the educational base of technical nursing practice to the ANA-NLN Coordinating Council. One concern was that issuing such a paper might detrimentally affect recruitment of new students into diploma programs defined as technical at just the point when "diploma education was finding it difficult to hold the line and produce nurses during a transition period until associate degree and baccalaureate programs are ready to do the total job."[37]

The NLN, which in 1970 accredited diploma programs in 556 institutions, wanted the ANA working paper to be written in such a way as not to imply that it was recommending the immediate cessation of these schools. The NLN board had earlier voted to work with the ANA and its Commission on Nursing Education, but clearly it would not back the ANA statement without regard for the position it took.

The Word *Technical*—Should It Have Been Divisive?

The word *technical* in the developing debate was emotionally charged largely because of a general misunderstanding of its origins. When in 1951 Montag issued the initial appeal for the preparation of a new kind of nurse in community colleges, she called that nurse "technical." As we have noted, the CRP itself assumed that the nursing role was not a single, monolithic one. Rather, it assumed that the various roles and functions of nursing practice could be differentiated: they do not compose separate universes, but instead lie along a continuum, "with professional at one end and technical at the other."[38]

But the word *technical* was used with special meaning by junior college educators in the late 1940s and 1950s. The scope of practice defined for the ADN by the CRP closely resembles the definition of technical or semiprofessional occupations by junior college educators at midcentury. The point is particularly important because the word was not being used in the way it was understood by the average person: *technical* was assumed to describe someone who is proficient, unusually skilled in the performance, especially in the manual performance, of procedures. The difference between the educators' and others' understanding of the connotations of the word, especially, gave rise to many problems. Not the least of these, according to Rines,[39] is that the technical, or AD, nurse possesses special proficiencies that are not, in fact, the central focus of the ADN curriculum.

Ruth Matheney, another early leader in the ADN movement, gave several definitions of technical occupations; these definitions reveal the uncertainty and lack of agreement about the meaning of the term *technical*.[40] She begins with Kenneth Beach's 1956 definition of a technical occupation as one that

1. requires skillful application of [a high degree of] specialized knowledge together with a broad understanding of operational procedures;
2. involves the frequent application of personal judgment;
3. [usually] deals with a variety of situations;
4. [and often] requires the supervision of others.

A technical occupation, Beach said, offers the opportunity for the worker to develop an ever-increasing personal control over the application of knowledge to work and usually requires fewer motor skills than a trade or a skilled occupation and less generalized knowledge than a profession.

The definition of technical occupations put forward by Norman C. Harris in 1966 revealed the gradually developing intellectual base for the concept. *Occupational education*, he said, refers to any and all education and training aimed at preparation for employment offered by the junior colleges, as distinguished from education in the liberal arts, the fine arts, or the humanities. Occupational education covers all levels —professional, technical, and skilled—of curricula for all fields of employment. Moreover, he said that semiprofessional education is represented by formal curricula leading to the associate degree and designed to prepare the student for employment in career fields recognized as nearly professional in status. Semiprofessional workers usually work in close cooperation with, perhaps under the direct supervision of, a professional worker.

However, *technical education*, Harris admitted, was a term just beginning to acquire meaning in 1966; there was no universally accepted definition. In his opinion, it was to be defined thus: technical education

1. is organized into two-year curriculums;
2. emphasizes work in the field of sciences and mathematics (though not necessarily);
3. gives much attention to technical knowledge and general education but also stresses practice and skill in the use of tools and instruments;
4. leads to competence in one of the technical occupations, and usually the granting of an associate degree;
5. includes a core of general education courses up to perhaps one-fourth of the total credit hours.[41]

The original ADN programs were developed on the basis of broad assumptions like these about the nature of semiprofessional and technical education. It was decided in the CRP that the new programs would prepare graduates to qualify for RN licensure (just as the graduates of the two other programs were) but also to meet the requirements for the associate degree, perform technical functions at the RN level, and be prepared to function as beginning practitioners and to *become* competent, *not* to be graduated fully competent. And although Mildred Montag has never faltered in the assertion that these remain the goals of the ADN, many in nursing education do not agree, and many ADN programs in the years since 1952 have in fact developed along other lines.

Matheney was also specific about what technical nurses should be expected to do. Technical nursing practice, in her view, is concerned primarily with the direct nursing of patients who present common, recurring nursing problems. The major focuses of technical nursing thus would be patients' physical comfort and safety, physiological malfunction, psychological and social difficulties, and rehabilitative needs. The technical nurse is responsible for providing not only nursing care but also medically delegated tasks. To fulfill these responsibilities, the technical nurse would need to use the problem-solving process to identify nursing problems, to plan nursing care, to evaluate the effectiveness of nursing intervention, and to revise nursing care plans as needed. These ideas were developed later in the project than were Montag's, but they belong to the same family of concepts.

Matheney's carefully detailed definition of technical nursing practice was widely used. However, some of the faculties developing new ADN programs and having little access to organized curriculum work evolved their own assumptions about technical nursing in isolation. As a consequence, the word *technical* often came to be associated with the "second best," and it has subsequently been discarded by many educators. In fact, the members of the NLN Council of Associate Degree Programs have voted to discard the word from their deliberations and publications. Others like Montag, however, still insist on the use of the word.

Hospital-based educators had great difficulty with the label "technical" and considered it second-best. When many moved from the NLN to the AHA's institutional membership for educational programs, one of their first acts was to relabel the diploma graduate as a professional nurse. But dissent over who was and who was not a nursing "professional" was gaining momentum. Proponents of the 1965 Position Paper of the ANA had labeled the diploma graduate "technical," not "professional." The words had become heavily loaded with political import, meanings that were not associated with the word *technical* when the ADN program was first designed.

Other Changes

The restructuring of the educational system to comply with the Position Paper called for additional changes that were to profoundly affect the course of nursing education in the near future.

First and foremost was the obvious need for community and statewide planning. During the 1968–1970 biennium the ANA Commission on Nursing Education spelled out criteria for all new nursing programs in a communication to state boards of nursing and to state nurses' associations. (During the late 1960s by far the most common new programs were, in fact, ADN programs.) The commission outlined the following minimum requirements: that the program be controlled by an educational institution—a college or university; that an adequate faculty, that is, people having graduate preparation in nursing and education, be available; that the program be provided with adequate financial support; that clinical learning laboratories for the projected number of students be provided. In the meantime, ANA delegates in convention expressed their continued support for the "sound and orderly transition of nursing education into institutions of higher learning."[42]

Throughout 1969 the ANA Commission on Nursing Education continued to express support for sound educational planning. It mailed letters to all state boards of nursing and state nurses' associations urging that they support the development of statewide plans. The NLN had long since called for community planning for nursing education, in 1962 urging state and local health, welfare, educational, and citizens' groups to plan cooperatively for an orderly transition from the diploma to the associate degree.[43] The general concern of all nursing leaders was that severe nursing shortages would result from the closure of diploma programs if another ready course of nurse manpower were not developed first.

Early on in the debate about the Position Paper the ANA board endorsed an ANA-NLN Joint Statement on Community Planning for Nursing Education. A second joint statement was endorsed in 1966.[44] The statement called for community planning marked by cooperation that would ensure an adequate supply of nurses. On 28 January 1967 the NLN issued another statement urging community planning to ward off acute nursing shortages, and it urged haste. Later that same year the league published its *Guidelines for Assessing the Nursing Education Needs of a Community*, which included both its 1962 statement and the 1966 joint statement with the ANA.[45]

Throughout the 1960s the NLN and the ANA began to lay the groundwork for educational restructuring. The NLN, for instance, focused considerable attention on career-pattern studies, a census of nurse faculty, and cost studies of baccalaureate, associate degree, and diploma programs. At the same time that the ANA Commission on Nursing Education began its work, 1967, the ANA-NLN Nursing Careers Program was initiated. There was a great hunger for hard facts: not only did planners need to know how many of each type of program existed year by year and how many students were enrolling and graduating from each type; they also needed to know what was happening to the nurses once they graduated. How many were leaving nursing, and why? How many returned to school for further education and training, and at what levels? Where was the nation educating nurses most effectively and with the greatest cost-effectiveness? Without facts, the future course would be uncharted. Without the facts, planning at any level would be difficult.

The policy of the NLN and the ANA boards was to continue to support all types of nursing programs, including LPN programs. Gwendoline MacDonald, president of the NLN, stated that, in keeping with the purposes of the league's program for school improvement, the organization had developed the following beliefs:

1. All programs should meet and maintain high standards.
2. All programs should move into institutions of higher education.
3. All programs should support educational planning at local, state, regional, and national levels to the end that a desirable balance of nursing personnel become available.
4. College and university nursing programs should be increased and strengthened to provide educators, administrators, clinical specialists, and others necessary for the future.[46]

An Attempt to Bring Order Out of Confusion

As the 1960s wore on, leaders in nursing became increasingly aware of the enormous complexity of the problems confronting the profession. Its educational disorder was part of the problem, to be sure, but only part. Somehow, it seemed illogical to assume that nursing educators alone could solve the problems. Indeed, some argued that nursing alone could not, that its problems were too rooted in larger social and health care issues for them to be solved in some sort of isolation.

In an attempt to bring a more comprehensive and encompassing vision to bear on the problems of nursing, the national nursing organizations established the National Commission for the Study of Nursing and Nursing Education in 1966. W. Allen Wallis, at the time president of the University of Rochester, headed the commission, and Jerome P. Lysaught was appointed the project director. This commission, whose formation had been recommended by the surgeon general's nursing consultants, would undertake studies and issue reports that would affect the thinking and work of many in nursing for years to come. Nursing education had more than its share of studies and evaluations, and the cynics might have been forgiven for heaving deep sighs at the formation of yet another study group. And yet, the work of an independent commission did hold hope for future unity and progress.

The ADN Movement: Issues at Maturity

The growth in the number of ADN programs continued unabated. In 1965, the year of the ANA Position Paper, there were 174 programs; five years later they numbered 444, an increase of 270.[1] By 1970, 27 percent of all American nurse graduates for the year were ADN graduates.[2] As the new ADN programs demonstrated their ability to educate students whose ability to pass licensure examinations matched that of other nursing programs, they gained credibility with government officials, foundation officers, and community college administrators.

The CRP had established the ADN program and demonstrated its viability. But what the project could not do, was not designed to do, was gain acceptance for ADN graduates in nursing educational and practice circles.

ADN graduates had difficulty earning legitimacy in American hospitals because they were prepared differently from the graduates of the traditional hospital-based program. It was never the intention of ADN educators to prepare a nurse ready to step into the work role of the staff nurse without first having an extensive orientation program. Novices required such assistance from their employers to assume the role expected of the hospital-based diploma graduate, who had more extensive hands-on experience and who was acquainted with the policies and procedures of the hospital from which she had graduated.

Misunderstandings during the 1960s about the work role for which the graduate was prepared were quite common. A doctoral dissertation at the time reported the lack of information administrators had about the new nurse and pointed out that as a consequence ADN graduates were assigned to responsibilities they were not ready to assume.[3] The result was their being labeled by many as incompetent or unsafe, and nursing practice administrators even questioned the ability of nurse educators to teach.

According to Robert Kinsinger, at the inception of the ADN program "and for many years following, a large percentage of practicing nurses, physicians, hospital administrators, and nurse educators in other types of nursing programs were opposed (sometimes confrontationally) to the advent of associate degree nursing education."[4]

A national debate ensued about the purposes of the ADN program. Internships and externships were recommended and in some hospitals were put in place. The addition of a third year to the ADN curriculum was a commonly voiced suggestion. ADN educators maintained that hospitals did not know how to use the AD nurse; practice administrators said that educators did not know how to teach novices.

A dialogue of national importance about the use of the technical nurse in hospitals began. Montag, Waters, and others wrote extensively about the skills and abilities the AD nurse did have on entry into practice,[5] but graduates continued to find themselves assigned as team leaders or charge nurses, roles for which they were unprepared when they first entered practice.

By the late 1960s the controversy spilled over into hospital and medical journals. Hospital-based programs found favor with physicians and hospital administrators, but nurses continued to argue for the movement of basic nursing education into junior and senior colleges and universities.

In 1974, 10.2 percent of all women graduates of American high schools were choosing nursing as a career—an all-time high.[6] (The appeal of a nursing career at this time may have been the indirect result of the strong support for nursing education that had been forthcoming from the federal government, support that was also at its peak at this time.) Consequently, the demand for admission to the ADN programs rose. By 1975 there were 618 ADN programs located in about 50 percent of American community colleges, a 10 percent growth rate since 1970.[7]

However, several community college administrators also had some doubts about the developing nursing programs. According to Robert Kinsinger, their second thoughts were based on several practical considerations: in most cases it was soon evident that nursing was the most costly program offered by the community college or at least among the top two or three offered at the institution. The complexity of providing a variety of laboratory settings and clinical experiences not under the direct control of the college provided an unparalleled challenge to administrators. In a good many instances, having to work with a state board of nursing for licensing their graduates was a unique and difficult experience for colleges. And finally, nursing faculty had no experience in the type of community college program in which they were teaching — their work was always a "first" into mostly unmapped territory.[8]

Social Change Causes a Change in Direction

The 1960s and early 1970s saw changes in American life and attitudes that would greatly affect nursing education. Not the least of these was the changing perception of the proper role of women in society, but also important was the increasing concern for equality, for the rights of minorities, for the rights of the consumer, and for increased social mobility by way of educational opportunity. Social pressures for change in all these would alter the course of nursing history.

In 1963 the NLN's Research and Studies Service launched a study that revealed little change in the percentage of black students admitted to schools of nursing over a twelve-year period: from 3.2 percent in 1951, when blacks made up 10 percent of the population, to 3.0 percent in 1963, when the black percentage of the population had risen to 10.5. Barbara Tate and Elizabeth Carnegie, who conducted the study, pointed to the devastating effect that the closing of predominantly black schools was having on overall black enrollment. They noted that from 1951 to 1963 ten such schools had closed their doors. Because 51.7 percent of black students admitted in 1962–1963 were enrolled in the 21 black schools then in existence, they reasoned that the closure of such programs would far more profoundly affect black admissions than would the law prohibiting racial segregation.[9] Both the ANA and the NLN took strong stands regarding the necessity for nondiscriminatory practices in nursing and nursing education. Clearly, though, there was also the need for strong action on the practical front.

In 1966 the Nurse Training Act was amended to provide nursing education opportunity grants for disadvantaged young people. Another amendment of 1966 directed to the nurse training authorities of the Public Health Service called for the creation of a program for nursing recruitment that would place emphasis on the recruitment of disadvantaged and minority students. In addition, Congress authorized additional money for loans for nursing students.[10] All these measures had the backing of the nursing organizations. Black enrollment in ADN and other nursing programs increased as a result of these measures.

Foundation support for AD nursing continued. In 1963 the NLN received an extension on a grant from the Sealantic Fund to provide for the sound development of ADN programs and to help those that were already established to evaluate their progress and to improve them. The funds were used to extend for three years the consultation services that the NLN had been providing to ADN administrators and to expand the services to include faculty members and community groups.[11] In 1967 the League received another grant from Sealantic to fund a comprehensive survey of the nation's ADN programs. By the summer of 1967 the nation's ADN programs numbered 281, and they graduated 4,654 new nurses that year.[12] Among the findings of the survey, according to Sylvia Lande, were these: (1) not all programs were operating on the basis of mandatory open admissions, (2) ADN curricula were characterized by broad groupings of subject matter, (3) the length of programs varied somewhat, and (4) only 3 percent of the graduates were continuing their formal education beyond this AD level.[13]

Also at issue was the continuation of the nation's practical nurse programs. The ANA was alarmed that the numbers of state-approved practical nursing programs had grown so rapidly, from 520 in 1958 to 1,252 in 1969. Enrollment in these programs was growing rapidly, too: from 17,925 in 1958 to 53,080 in 1969.[14] The ANA proposed that the profession work "systematically" to facilitate the replacement of programs for practical nursing with programs for "beginning technical nursing practice in junior colleges."[15] Career-mobility programs for working women would be needed to put this recommendation into place.

The movement toward career mobility both for LPNs and for RNs gained momentum in the 1960s. Not only the associate degree but the baccalaureate degree was made more accessible. An important assumption of the CRP was that the ADN program was complete—a terminal program. It would prepare a nurse for "immediate employment," and no further education would be necessary. But the assumption was to become untenable in a society concerned with equality of opportunity, access to education, and social mobility by way of that opportunity.

Initially, Montag believed that ADN and BSN programs could not and should not be articulated. As she perceived them, the purposes, curricular content, and teaching methods of the two programs were so different that it would not be possible to apply a ladder concept of curriculum development to them. She describes the CRP and other early ADN programs as "content with being what they were intended to be—complete within themselves, possessing an integrity of their own." Even now, in the 1980s, she suggests that

> if too much attention is paid to articulation with the baccalaureate program both programs will suffer. So much emphasis on mobility leads me to suspect a less than complete confidence in, or acceptance of, the technical program, and ultimately in the differentiation of functions. If this is so, then we have returned to the idea that "a nurse is a nurse is a nurse." When AD programs were still in their pilot stage, we stated that we believed this would be the only formal education for most of the students, but that no barriers would or should stand in the way of those who sought to change their career goals. I see no reason today to change this belief.[16]

The Reform Movement Continues

Stepping into the controversy with a soothing effect was nursing's reaction to the reforms that were implicit in the recommendations of the National Commission on Nursing and Nursing Education, known more commonly as the Lysaught study.

Several specific recommendations of the commission had a more direct bearing on the ADN movement. Four, in particular, prompted action that would greatly affect the two-year programs. The commission had recommended (1) statewide planning for the number and distribution of nurse education programs, (2) interinstitutional studies of nursing curricula, (3) career mobility for individual nurses, and (4) the unity of nursing practice and education in working toward the same goals of improved patient care. Each of these would find expression in action or studies that would shape ADN education for a number of years to come.

Until the Lysaught commission's report, little emphasis had been placed on the progression of the nursing student from one program to the next higher one in nursing. In fact, nursing educators other than Montag believed that the ADN curriculum was not enough like the baccalaureate to serve as a basis for progression from the ADN to the BSN. Students wishing to obtain the BSN degree needed to start their postsecondary education over again, according to this line of thought. It was assumed by some in baccalaureate education that the curricula of the two nursing programs were not related, that they occupied two separate universes. In point of fact, educators did little to encourage the graduates of ADN programs to continue on to the baccalaureate level, and at this time only about 10 percent of the ADN graduates were pursuing the higher degree.

But the commission recommended the development of an education system for nursing that would dovetail with the practice arena on the basis of the differences in practice to be expected from the two- and the four-year graduates. The commissioners assumed that students should be able to progress from the lower-level programs to the upper-level programs without difficulty. What was most important in this thinking, from the standpoint of ADN education, was the assumption that the practice of the ADN graduate was different from that of graduates of the other programs—differentiated practice having been the cornerstone upon which the entire ADN movement had been built. That cornerstone found implicit reaffirmation in the Lysaught commission's goals.

In response to the commission's recommendation that interinstitutional studies of nursing curricula be conducted, the Kellogg Foundation funded three such efforts. One was conducted at the Southern Regional Education Board in Atlanta; one was based in Orange County, California; and a third, the SNAP project, was located in New Mexico. Each of these studies identified the work role of the nurse in hospitals and other health care agencies at the entry level and assigned various tasks to educators working in the nursing curriculum at various levels of the educational system. Recommendations for career mobility through interinstitutional planning was at the forefront of each study's report.

Precisely what was to be expected of the graduates of each of the nursing programs—the ADN, the diploma, and the BSN—was clearly spelled out; these expectations were labeled "competencies," as was then the vogue in educational literature. The curricula were teased apart, and the competencies were grouped according to their use in what were labeled "primary," "secondary," and "tertiary" levels of health care. Within this scheme, the content of the ADN program remained just as it had been outlined and defined in the 1950s. The content of the baccalaureate and graduate-level programs were clearly detailed as different from the content of the ADN program, particularly in the areas of primary and tertiary care. As called for in the commission's original recommendations, the studies clearly delineated the respective curricular objectives, alternatives, and sequences in each type of nursing program.

In the late 1960s career mobility was an idea in the ascendancy, and articles began to appear in the literature describing advanced standing in the next highest program, plans developed within and between programs and institutions to facilitate advanced education for the ADN and the hospital-based nurse. Even before the commission's report was issued, Rena Boyle in 1966 had first described the three-tiered program developed at the University of Nebraska to facilitate career advancement.[17]

In 1967 the ANA had published a brochure, inspired by the Position Paper, entitled "Avenues for Continued Learning." It encouraged continuing and advanced formal education for all practicing nurses, without regard to their previous preparation.[18] The momentum was propelled forward when in 1968 the Kellogg Foundation funded a workshop entitled "Toward Differentiation of Associate and Baccalaureate Nursing Education and Practice." It was held in August for the benefit of directors and instructors in ADN programs in northern California and was led by Mary Searight, who later developed a "second step" program for RNs who wished to continue their education.[19]

In 1970 Laura Dustan described efforts in Iowa to develop lower-division courses acceptable to BSN programs for transfer of credit. By 1975 a statewide plan for career mobility in Oklahoma was put forward.[20]

During the time of these advances, the Kellogg Foundation also funded the New York External Degree Program, which was a giant step for nursing into nontraditional education.[21] Its fully developed associate degree program, which was an evaluative rather than an instructional plan, was to cause an outpouring of emotional opinion about such testing of nursing content. Was it safe to qualify nurses by testing them after independent study? Would the state boards of nursing consider such tests valid for licensure? Was this national program a threat to the local junior colleges?

By 1972 the NLN had prepared an anthology entitled *The Associate Degree Program—A Step to the Baccalaureate Degree in Nursing.*[22] And in 1974 the short- and long-range goals of the NLN's open curriculum project, a major endeavor, were announced.[23]

The National Commission believed that continued federal assistance and private grants and endowments were necessary for the growth and development of nursing as a profession. In fact, they considered additional federal assistance essential, in light of the fact that their lack of endowments left nursing schools with marginal financing—a situation that was in stark contrast to that of other professional schools, which commonly benefited from generous endowments.

Although recommendations of the Lysaught commission were more forward-looking than those of the Brown study of 1948, they were in line with the thrust of the earlier report. As an example, the commission recommended that diploma programs seek degree-granting status, adding the assertion that their very survival rested on their obtaining such status. It also recommended improved reward systems for practicing nurses, better recruitment strategies, and greater representation on national and regional health policy and planning councils.

In 1981 Lysaught published a report of a longitudinal follow-up study of the recommendations of the National Commission for the Study of Nursing and Nursing Education.[24] At about the same time, two more studies of nursing and nursing education having national importance were being conducted, to be formally reported in 1983. The first was sponsored by the National Commission on Nursing, an independent commission sponsored by the American Hospital Association, the Hospital Research and Educational Trust, and the American Hospital Supply Corporation. The second study was sponsored by the Institute of Medicine of the National Academy of Sciences.

In 1981 the initial report and preliminary recommendations of the National Commission on Nursing were published, and the summary report and recommendations were issued in 1983. The commission was charged with (1) analyzing the nurse's work environment, (2) identifying the effects of professional nursing issues on nursing practice, (3) exploring the incentives to enter and practice nursing, (4) analyzing the ways nursing education, practice, and research interrelate in practice, and (5) planning methods to enhance the status of nurses through the study of the role of the nurse in health care.[25]

The study by the Institute of Medicine was "prompted by controversy in the late 1970s as to whether further substantial federal outlays for nursing education would be needed to assure an adequate supply of nurses."[26] Over an eighteen-year period beginning in 1965, more than $1.6 billion had been appropriated under the various Nurse Training Acts. The year 1983 saw the publication of the final report of the Institute's study.

The three studies, despite their differing orientations and bases of support, arrived at strikingly similar conclusions on a number of points that were highly important to the ADN movement. All three endorsed greater unity of nursing education and nursing service; in effect, all three noted the gap between the two sectors in nursing that had developed over the years. All three focused on the need to improve the nursing curriculum, though each emphasized different issues: the Lysaught commission, interinstitutional studies; the AHA, the development of a common body of knowledge and skills uniting all nursing programs; the Institute of Medicine, the need for more content in geriatrics. All three insisted on the need for increased recruiting into nursing, the Institute of Medicine emphasizing especially the need to attract more minority and nontraditional students into the field. All three promoted the concept of career mobility within the field, which rests on the efficient articulation of educational programs of differing lengths and benefits from fuller development of nontraditional and outreach programs. The latter point was emphasized by the Institute of Medicine. All three directed attention to the need for better rewards for those who make nursing their life's work—rewards being not only better pay but other material benefits as well as status. The Institute spoke of restructuring the rewards system in nursing. Closely allied with such improvements were issues highlighted by the Lysaught and Nursing Commission studies: increasing the voice of nursing in the making of policy at both the national and the regional levels and offering better recognition of the nurse's contribution to the nation's overall health care.

All three studies asserted the need for increased federal funding for nursing education. The Institute of Medicine specifically recommended the creation of a Center for Nursing Research, greater support for graduate nursing education, student loans, and support directed to meet particular shortages as they develop. All three emphasized the need for more and better nursing research.

The Lysaught commission and the Nursing Commission agreed on a number of points the Institute of Medicine did not cover: they endorsed better articulation of programs and the consequent increase in the number of nurses progressing to baccalaureate and graduate levels of training; they also emphasized the need to make better use of staff nurses by placing the responsibility for non-nursing functions on other staff members and providing better support systems for nursing staff.

Finally, the Lysaught commissioners and the Institute of Medicine agreed that planning for nursing education was essential and that it needed to be coordinated at the state level, using such bodies, for example, as state master planning committees.[27]

ADN Education at the Age of Twenty

The costs of health care rose precipitously in the late 1960s and early 1970s. The percentage of the GNP spent for health care rose a full percentage point from 1965 to 1969 (5.9 to 6.9).[1] In 1969 the number of full-time-equivalent nurses working in the labor force had increased by 55,000 since 1966, and approximately two of every three licensed nurses were participating, but even this level of participation was not enough to meet the demand.[2] The hospital RN vacancy rate was down to 11.2 percent from the 18.1 percent rate in 1967, and yet still more nurses were needed.[3] In 1969, 6 percent of female high school students were choosing nursing as a career, a rate increased from 5.3 percent in 1966, but not enough inactive nurses were returning to work to compensate for the 11,172 RNs serving in the military in Vietnam.[4]

In the mid-1970s the Division of Nursing surveyed 10,000 inactive RNs to learn the reasons for their inactivity in nursing. The reasons the nurses gave for dropping out of practice were that they were needed at home, that they had been unable to arrange for child care, that salaries were too low, and that working hours were unacceptable.[5]

Federal Responses to Nursing Shortages and the ADN Movement

Concern among federal officials about the nursing shortage remained high, and considerable effort was made to ascertain the facts about nursing manpower and to use these to arrive at reliable projections of future needs.[6] The year 1971 saw the culmination of a four-year study conducted by Stewart Altman and underwritten by the Division of Nursing; the results were published under the title *Present and Future Supply of Registered Nurses*. In examining the economic variables affecting nurse supply, Altman collected annual data to 1969; his projections covered 1970–1980. Among other things, his study revealed the decided shift of students from diploma to ADN and BSN programs.[7]

Hearings on new legislation directed toward a solution to the crisis in the education of health care professionals were held during April before both houses of Congress. Because on 30 June 1971 the Health Manpower Act of 1971 would expire, and with it the funds for nursing education it had provided, Congress passed and the president signed a temporary measure to extend the act's student loan and scholarship loan program until further legislation could be enacted. Finally, without ceremony, the Nurse Training Act of 1971 was signed by the president in the late fall.[8]

Equally important for AD nursing education, perhaps more so, was the provision under the 1971 Nurse Training Act for federal funding to nursing schools on the basis of capitation. This was the first time federal funds had been made available on this basis to nursing. Financial distress grants, start-up grants, and recruitment funding were also provided for under the new legislation.[9]

The Nursing Student Loan Program, which assisted students enrolled in ADN and other programs, now included 943 schools and programs on its list, an increase of 121 percent since 1965, just six years. The Division of Nursing distributed $34 million to 1,098 nursing education programs in 1971–1972. Capitation grants were set at $250 for each full-time student enrolled at the undergraduate level, and $500 for each graduate student; $100 was available for each student enrolled that went beyond the school's annual projection of number of students expected.[10] Such funding was critically important for many programs: consider the impact for a school enrolling, say, 115 students—an additional $28,750 for the program budget. The relative importance of the capitation grants to the nursing schools was calculated by determining the percentage of average net educational expenditures by a program that the capitation funds represented; in 1972–1973 the federal funds represented anywhere from 13 percent (for ADN programs) to 22 percent (diploma programs). These percentages implied a fairly high degree of dependence on capitation funding, but the nursing schools were less dependent than were programs in other fields: 30 percent in veterinary medicine, 41 percent in osteopathy, 38 percent in dentistry, and 29 percent in medicine.[11]

From 1965 to 1971 the federal program had provided more than

$380 million to nursing education, and the impact of such funding was obvious. Graduates from nursing programs increased during this period, from 34,686 to 47,000. About one-half of the expenditures under the program directly benefited students: $123 million for loans and scholarships, $68 million for traineeships to 48,000 persons, $97 million for construction that resulted in space for 6,200 new students, and $34 million for 343 special project grants directly affecting students. In addition, ten nonprofit agencies received $1 million for recruiting and retraining nursing personnel.[12] Both the ANA and the NLN appeared at the hearings during April 1971 to press for further government backing of nursing education.[13]

Indeed, so important had lobbying in Washington become for the nursing profession that in January of 1971 the ANA moved its Government Relations Department offices to the nation's capital. And in 1972 the Nurses for Political Action, Inc., was established and soon became affiliated with the ANA. Its goals were to influence national policy in health affairs, to campaign for nurse representation on committees designing legislation, and recognition for nurses in primary practice working for a fee.[14]

National politics were now making an impact on nursing education. The early legislation thrusting the federal government into direct funding of nursing education had been enacted under Kennedy and Johnson; the measures were expressions of the social policy and resultant programs of those two administrations. By 1971, however, the Nixon administration had been in office for nearly a full term, and it was gearing up for a new election in 1972. The administration was opposed to any expansion of the programs under the Nurse Training Act. A report on the act, *The Progress Report on Nurse Training—1970,* which had been mandated by Congress, was published, though given to Congress unobtrusively and in an abridged form. By the end of the 1971 fiscal year the Division of Nursing faced a backlog in $20 million of approved but unfunded applications for construction grants. In all, thirty-four nursing schools were awaiting funds, fifteen of them associate degree programs.[15]

Nixon's landslide victory at the polls in 1972 gave him the mandate he needed to launch a determined effort to dismantle the program of federal aid to nursing and other similar programs. A large portion of the appropriation for fiscal year 1973 was legally impounded, for a total loss to the program of $73 million.[16] The Division of Nursing itself was protected from being dismantled only by a series of continuing resolutions by Congress.

In response, the NLN in 1973 filed suit against Roy Ash, director of the Office of Management and Budget, and Caspar Weinberger, secretary of the Department of Health, Education, and Welfare. The suit was intended to compel the award of $21.7 million budgeted for capitation grants. The league charged that the administration's impoundment of appropriated funds was illegal and that it violated the intent of Congress. On 29 June 1973 the U.S. District Court granted a temporary restraining order, and on 10 July a preliminary injunction was granted in favor of the NLN. Six months later a federal judge ordered the release of the impounded funds to the nursing schools that were league members. An additional $52 million was released later.[17]

The reduced role of the federal government in the nation's health affairs was spelled out by Weinberger. He specified that the government would support services to increase the access to care, research that had broad national application, preventive health and consumer measures that could best be achieved through collective action, and it would offer limited support to structural changes in the health care system and to health manpower activities. He added that the government would provide for direct medical care only as a last resort to citizens whose right to care was recognized in law or whose need was especially acute because of the failure of traditional means for providing health services.[18]

Also under the new austerity program, the Division of Nursing was transferred to the newly created Health Resources Administration. The decentralization of its services, also mandated from above, nearly destroyed the division.[19]

Despite the administration's effort to keep the lid on federal funding to nursing education, federal funding reached its highest level in 1974. Appropriations were for $313.5 million under the Nurse Training Act, and $135.6 million to help resolve the growing health manpower problem. The impact of federal funding from 1965 to 1974 was considerable: more than $154 million had been awarded to nursing schools for student loan programs, and 224 construction grants had gone to 94 baccalaureate and graduate programs, 79 ADN programs, and 51 diploma programs. Overall, the federal funds had allowed the creation of 11,000 new spaces for nursing students.[20]

The Nurse Training Act of 1971 had established financial distress grants. Awards under this program were designed to cover the costs of emergency damages (e.g., those occurring during floods), of uncertainty of program quality for a limited period, and of special efforts by a program (e.g., to upgrade or expand). In 1973 a total of 125 of these grants for $8.3 million were made to 35 diploma programs, 38 ADN programs, and 52 baccalaureate programs. In 1973–1974 awards totaled $1.4 million, a sizable reduction.[21]

But projections for continued federal assistance to nursing education were becoming extremely bleak. The ANA and other national organizations sent distress calls to nurses throughout the country, seeking their support for reinvigorated lobbying in Washington and asking them to push for change by lobbying their own representatives. The predictions were that all support for nursing research would be ended; traineeship support would be terminated; loans and scholarships for nursing students would be cut from $19.5 million to $11 million, nearly in half; capitation grants would be first cut in half and then terminated; and there would be no funding for recruitment programs, financial distress situations, start-ups of new programs, or new special programs. The apparent plan was to return as much decision making as possible to the local institution and to state and local government.[22]

It was predicted that federal funding would drop from the nearly $60 million provided in fiscal year 1973 to $52 million in 1974, on its way to nearly complete phasing out of federal support. Under the proposed revision of health manpower training programs, the special categorical funding for nurse training would be abolished. The total health manpower training budget request for the fiscal year 1975 was $369 million, fully $198 million less than for the preceding year. Funds for nurse training were to reach only $45 million.[23]

By lobbying very hard, the ANA, the NLN, and other nursing organizations were able to persuade Congress to restore the $146 million budgeted for fiscal year 1974, which was the last of the three years covered under the Nurse Training Act of 1971. On 30 November 1974 the Interstate and Foreign Commerce Committee reported out a bill known as the Nurse Training Act of 1974, which represented few changes from the 1971 act. Although the bill passed both houses of Congress, Ford gave it a pocket veto on 3 January 1975. By enacting continuing resolutions, Congress extended budget authorizations from 1974 into fiscal year 1975. And the struggle continued. The report *Nurse Training—1974*, which as in 1970 was mandated under the law, was presented to Congress, but (as in 1970) as inconspicuously as possible, in abridged form.[24]

The nursing organizations continued to plead before congressional committees for the extension of the basic framework of the Nurse Training Act of 1971. Witnesses for the administration maintained that little aid was actually needed. Stuart Altman, deputy assistant secretary of HEW and author of the first manpower study in nursing, declared, "We are getting close to where there is no longer a shortage of nurses," and he claimed that sixteen states even had a surplus.[25] The hospital vacancy rates for RNs were on the rise—9.3 percent in 1971, 10 percent the next year, and 10.5 percent in 1973—despite the fact that the labor force participation rate for RNs had now risen to 70.5 percent.[26]

Early in 1975 the AHA surveyed all fifty state hospital associations to evaluate the shortage of RNs in hospitals. A shortage of nurses in health care facilities in 36 states, or nearly three-fourths of the country, was reported. "Of the 14 states in which no overall statewide shortage was apparent, a majority indicated serious shortages of available registered nurses in certain areas, especially areas of rural and low-income populations." AHA officials reported that hospitals were stepping up their recruitment programs, using LPNs in the place of RNs, and employing foreign nurses to fill the gaps.[27] Furthermore, during the next few years the RN vacancy rates in hospitals rose, from 11.5 percent in 1975 to 14 percent in 1979, just four years later.[28] This number was down from the high of the early 1960s, but it matched the alarming numbers that had been reported during the mid-1950s. The facts strongly suggested that despite the repeated denials of officials of the Nixon and Ford administrations that any nursing shortages threatened, shortages would indeed continue to plague the health care system.

In 1975 the Nurse Training Act of 1971, already extended for one year, was due to expire, and Congress was deliberating the terms of a new act, the Nurse Training Act of 1975, to extend coverage through fiscal year 1978. The opposition was sharply critical of the program. The Ford administration was adamantly opposed to what it called unnecessary and inflationary expenditures on health care education, and many senators and representatives argued that the federal government had been propelled into support of nursing education only to meet a temporary crisis.

The proposed legislation authorized lower funding for capitation grants than in previous years, but when the House health subcommittee increased grants for ADN programs, triggering pressure from proponents of baccalaureate and diploma programs for like increases, the administration reasserted its intention to veto the measure. The authorization levels in the bill that was finally reported out of committee were indeed lower than in preceding years: down $75 million in FY 1976, $50 million in FY 1977, and $25 million in FY 1978. Moreover, support was to shift gradually away from traditional nursing education and toward more innovative programs.

Ford did veto the bill, but Congress quickly overrode the veto. The new Nurse Training Act continued the existing traineeship programs for 1975 and authorized $60 million over fiscal years 1976–1978.[29] These same years saw drastic reductions in the support of the direct operation of the Division of Nursing. Its reduced percentage of the overall budget, its greatly reduced staff, and its decentralization during these years meant that it "had virtually been bled to death."[30]

Projections of the number of nurses needed to meet future manpower demands were sorely needed by 1976, some nine years after the Altman study had begun. In 1976 the Division of Nursing commissioned two manpower studies of nursing, each of which employed a method that would be widely used for the next decade. One, the historical trend-based model, estimated future requirements for RNs by extending current trends in the use of RN services and resources into the future, adjusting the estimates on the basis of assumptions about how system trends might affect these nursing trends. The other, the criteria-based model, examined what future requirements for nurses might be if given health care goals were used to determine needed levels of service. The latter model had been developed by WICHEN in the 1970s and was widely supported by the nursing community. The models were maintained and updated over the years in work farmed out to WICHEN and a private group in Boston by the staff of the Bureau of the Health Professions. The results of both models have been reviewed and revised to take into account new strategies being employed by the health care system that might affect the system's requirements for nursing personnel.[31] Consequently, two reports are issued to Congress each year, one emanating from the Nurse Training Act and the other, on the distribution of requirements for nurses, emanating from the projections determined by each model.

By 1976, with the advent of a new administration under Jimmy Carter, federal officials were predicting a surplus of nurses, or at least a balance between supply and demand by 1979, and for the foreseeable future. The budget for the Nurse Training Act was reduced, financial distress grants were discontinued, and an income means test was added for student loans.

The Organizational Debate Continues

The professional nursing organizations continued to be highly concerned with the educational issues. In June of 1975 the ANA Commission on Nursing Education issued *Standards for Nursing Education*.[32] Although the commission that year had developed new definitions of technical and professional nursing, the ANA board tabled the commission's motion to have these definitions used by the association in its official business.

Opposition to the 1965 Position Paper was gaining momentum. Many nurses resented the technical label. Diploma programs were closing at a very rapid rate. In 1970, 47 percent of all nursing programs were hospital based, but by 1975 so many diploma programs had closed that they now represented only 31 percent of all programs. Since the adoption of the Position Paper, the number of hospital programs had dropped from 821 to 428. At the same time, ADN programs had gained ground dramatically, rising from 174 programs (15 percent) in 1965 to 618 (45 percent) just ten years later.[33] Nevertheless, the overwhelming majority of nurses on hospital staffs were graduates of diploma programs. Thus, although the shift was clearly away from the hospital program, it was not as much toward the baccalaureate as reformers desired.[34] The pressure to name the four-year degree as the minimum for entry into *professional* practice was fueling an increasingly heated argument within the ranks of nursing. It mattered little whether the division was described as following the old practice-academe split, or as marking a new one between types of programs; the division was deep, and it boded ill for nursing as a whole.

Then, in 1976 the New York State Nurses' Association (NYSNA) lobbied for legislation to implement the ANA Position Paper. The legislation would require the possession of the BSN for entry into the professional practice of nursing in New York State. In April of 1976 the ANA Commission on Nursing Education appointed a task force to examine the issues raised by the NYSNA effort to translate the Position Paper into law. The task force included representatives of the AACN, the National Federation of Licensed Practical Nurses, and the National Student Nurses' Association.

Reaction at the national level came almost immediately. In June 1976 the House of Delegates of the ANA voted to convene a national conference of appropriate representatives who would write a statement for the ANA on the entry into nursing practice. The purpose of the conference was to allow debate of the issues, discussion of ways to implement the recommendations of the original Position Paper, and to propose plans for further action on the entry issues.[35]

The conference was held in February 1978—in Kansas City in the middle of a blizzard. Those who managed to attend (440 had planned to take part) worked within the framework of three resolutions adopted the preceding June by the House of Delegates, which charged the conference with these tasks: (1) to identify and title two categories (levels, or types) of nursing practice; (2) to establish a mechanism for deriving competency statements regarding each; and (3) to increase the options for career mobility in nursing.[36]

The conference participants produced three resolutions, which were adopted by the House of Delegates at the 1978 ANA convention. These resolutions were as follows:

1. That the ANA ensure two categories of nursing practice to be identified and titled by 1980, that by 1985, the minimum preparation for entry into professional nursing practice be the baccalaureate in nursing. The ANA was to work with state and other nurses' organizations to identify and define the two categories as well as national guidelines for implementation, and report back by 1980.
2. That the ANA establish a mechanism for deriving a comprehensive statement of competencies for the two categories of nursing practice by 1980.
3. That the ANA actively support increased access to high-quality career mobility programs that use flexible approaches for individuals seeking academic degrees.

What was new in these resolutions that was not contained in the 1965 Position Paper? They presented deadlines: 1980 for naming and describing the two categories of practice already in place, and 1985 for implementing them. And yet, the differentiation of nursing roles in the workplace, which is inherent in the development of the ADN movement, had not yet been accepted by the majority of nurses. Implicit in the 1978 resolutions was the need to differentiate roles and credentialing for the baccalaureate and the less-than-baccalaureate-trained nurse. But the resolutions provided no specifics, no direction as to how this differentiation was to be accomplished. There was no statement whether it should be accomplished by licensing, certification, or differentiated job descriptions for workers.

The resolutions also changed the terminology that had been used in the 1965 Position Paper. The framers sought consensus and compromise through the careful use of language. The term *level* was rejected and *category* substituted. The term *professional* was retained, but the other category was left without a title, the term *technical* having attracted much negative response. That associate degree education should be the requirement for the untitled category was reaffirmed.

The resolutions did differ markedly from the Position Paper in one important way: the third resolution legitimized career mobility, which the Position Paper of 1965 had not done. But attitudes were changing, and increasing numbers of nursing educators were coming to believe that the ADN and the BSN programs might not be so totally unrelated after all. Events in the real world were certainly moving nursing education in the direction of greater coherence and articulation. More and more graduates of ADN programs were returning to school to complete the bachelor's, and about the same time in California, legislators passed a law permitting BSN students to write the licensing examination after only thirty-six months, or three years, in the baccalaureate program.

In February of 1978, two years after its push to change the law in New York, the NYSNA approached the ANA board to request its endorsement of the state group's efforts to continue to implement the 1965 ANA Position Paper in New York. The board voted to endorse their efforts to "implement baccalaureate preparation for entry into professional nursing practice and associate degree preparation for nursing at the assisting level," and to provide licensure for each to enter practice. A few months later, in May, the ANA's Commission on Nursing Education asked the board for clarification, apparently puzzled by the board's endorsement of the New York move in the light of its prior commitment to the task force on entry into practice. Had the board preempted the work of the group?

In June the board responded, defining their duties to provide direction in response to action taken by the delegates. The board pointed out that the ANA had in place two of the stands called for, namely, the Position Paper endorsing the concept of two levels of practice and acceptance of the practice of licensing nurses before entry into the work world.

The ANA, in short, was already in support of licensure for two types of nurses. But the board also noted the possibility of the ANA's changing position, depending on the outcomes of the work of the task force on entry into practice.[37]

While debate over the issues continued to rage, at nursing meetings all over the nation and in the pages of nursing journals, the official stance of the ANA remained on hold. At the 1980 convention the House of Delegates, by consensus, agreed to delay a decision on titles until 1982, when the ANA Commission on Education would have completed its report, which would offer a comprehensive statement on the work role. Further progress was stalled as state nurses' associations struggled to reach consensus. The 1978 Action Survey by the ANA indicated that only eight states had taken formal positions on entry into practice, and only three—New York, Ohio, and Tennessee—had formulated positions that called for two levels of nursing practice, at the associate degree and baccalaureate levels. It appeared that the profession would not be able to meet the deadlines set in the original three resolutions.

In the meantime, the NLN board of directors in February 1976 approved the open curriculum concept, in effect putting its stamp of approval on the concept of career mobility. It, too, had a subgroup working on differentiating the competencies of the graduates of the different educational programs; the report of that task force was issued in final form in 1979.[38] The document delineated the competencies of graduates of LPN, ADN, diploma, and baccalaureate programs and included a review of the literature, methodologies, findings, and recommendations of other groups working on the same task.

In February 1981 the NLN adopted a statement on nursing education that supported all educational programs in nursing, in response, it said, to the social reality. But in February 1982, the board of directors issued a new position statement, naming the baccalaureate degree as minimum preparation for professional nursing practice.[39]

Thus, in 1982, seventeen years after the Position Paper was issued by the ANA, and thirty-four years after the Brown Report, which had recommended collegiate education for all nurses, both leading national nursing organizations were in official agreement: the professional nurse was the nurse who had received her nursing education in a four-year collegiate program. The associate degree also had a firm place in a level or category of nursing practice that was now unnamed. The road to the positions the national leaders were taking seemed long. Only time would tell whether nurses could find their way.

Nursing education in the mid-1970s was well on its way to an open system of education that would promote goals that individual nurses could choose. Educational opportunities for advancement were now offered at times and places convenient to those wishing to move forward. The ADN movement had been a major catalyst in this accomplishment.

The Kellogg Project:

The Work Role of the AD Nurse

By 1977 the ADN, more than any other educational program in nursing, had moved nursing education solidly into the general system of education. In just two decades the number of ADN programs had grown to 656, nearly half of the total number of nurse education programs in the country.[1] Graduates of these programs were 47 percent of the total number of graduates that year.[2] Approximately 52 percent of all American junior colleges had ADN programs. And yet, despite the vigor of the ADN program, the controversy surrounding it would not die. Its accomplishments were just not enough for the growing number of nurses who wanted at least the baccalaureate as the first professional degree. Both national nursing organizations had so named the baccalaureate, designating 1982 as the year for achieving this goal within the profession. The number of BSN programs had indeed grown during the 1970s, but by 1977 they still constituted but 30 percent of the total. Nevertheless, the desire for the baccalaureate as the basic program remained strong in nursing circles. And as a consequence, some AD nurses and the faculty who prepared them began to feel undervalued and unappreciated.

Theoretically, according to the original assumptions about technical nursing practice, ADN graduates needed the supervision of the better educated or the more experienced nurse, but in practice the supervision envisioned was not always present. The AD nurse had not become the assistant to the professional, as had been assumed by many. RNs were employed by most hospitals to perform the same work role, regardless of their educational preparation. All were paid the same salary. Differences in the practice of nurses who had graduated from various educational programs were difficult to measure, and many early studies of these differences neglected the cognitive aspects of the work role.

Not only did most hospitals ignore the differences between RNs from ADN programs and RNs from BSN programs, they also wanted all the nurses they hired to perform at the level of the experienced worker shortly after first being employed. This expectation had not been unrealistic at a time when most new staff nurses were graduates of a diploma program who elected to work at the home hospital; they and the hospital benefited from the built-in orientation supplied in effect by the program. But the ADN graduate came to the hospital as a true novice, having fewer clinical practice hours than her counterpart in the traditional diploma program. Consequently, though the new ADN graduate possessed a knowledge base that was the same or better than that of other new graduates, she required a longer orientation program and an added opportunity to practice procedural skills.

Nonetheless, as the 1980s began, ADN graduates were still being criticized for their lack of clinical abilities upon initial employment. The literature complained of their inability to make decisions, to set goals in priority order, to care for the number of patients required to maintain the staffing pattern planned by nurse administrators (see, e.g., items listed in the subject index under "ADN graduate" in the companion volume to this one). The policy question for nurse educators was, What is enough for the novice nurse to know and to do in her beginning job? Also, who is responsible for the development of the novice, and to support her as she learns on the job? Where does the educator's job end and the in-service hospital educator's begin? Should there be joint efforts of service and education to bridge the gap between the service's expectations and the graduate's abilities? Should these take the form of preceptorships, extern and intern programs, or clinical clerkships?

The hospital environment changed rapidly in the 1970s and 1980s. Acuity levels rose, diagnostic related groups (DRGs) necessitated early discharge, home care became more preeminent in health care delivery, and ambulatory surgery and care were promoted to save costs. Hospital patients were acutely and critically ill, and their care was becoming more complex and difficult. Nursing *turn-off* and *burnout* became commonplace words in hospitals. The "glitter and glamor" of high-technology care gave way to real questions about the parameters of the ADN program: Was the ADN curriculum adequate in its present form to prepare nurses for the realities of acute hospital care?

Many barriers to the solution of these policy questions were in evidence. Little communication passed between nursing service personnel and nurse educators. No differentiated job descriptions existed.

AD nurses were expected on initial appointment to perform the same tasks, make the same decisions, and walk in the same shoes as the baccalaureate graduates. The evaluation of nursing staff in hospitals was based on this uniformity of expectations; indeed, little performance evaluation was being done. A nurse of any preparatory level could be employed in any part of the hospital without specialty training or preparation. Career ladders based on clinical proficiency as a criterion for promotion were seldom used.

As a consequence, the role assigned the AD nurse became increasingly complex. Nurses assigned to general medical-surgical units were faced with job responsibilities for which they were minimally prepared. Excellent two-year programs were faced with deciding which portion of an expanding curriculum to include. AD nurses complained of the complexity of the staff nurse role on medical-surgical units and elected specialty practice in various ICU and neonatal units, despite the fact that there was no specialty training at the AD level.

The skills and abilities for which the baccalaureate graduate was prepared went unused while AD graduates were asked to perform in complex nursing situations beyond their abilities. Demonstration units to show the potential for a complementary relationship between the two did not exist.

Moreover, approximately half the teachers in ADN programs were academically unprepared for their jobs. Persons working in community colleges were not knowledgeable about the mission of the college, the curriculum suitable for AD nurses, and the differences in roles between BSN and ADN graduates.

Novice program planning was in disarray. A few hospitals had orientation units or externship and internship programs, but many struggled along with situations that left novice nurses unsatisfied and uncertain about what was expected of them. In-service education staffs were faced with increasing complexities in planning adequate staff development programs. Faculties were occasionally unsafe in specific clinical areas, and something more was needed to ensure patient safety.

Another serious shortage of nurses would further complicate the situation. Demoralization would surely increase. Novice nurses without mentors or adequate supervision might decide to drop out. By the early 1980s the quality of the pool of applicants to nursing programs was declining noticeably, and many feared it would decline further. Changes were not only desirable, they were necessary.

The Kellogg Foundation as Catalyst for Action

To address the continuing controversy, partially focused on issues of titling and credentialing in nursing, the W. K. Kellogg Foundation again stepped in and in 1977 convened an ad hoc advisory committee to consult with foundation officers.[3] The group was asked to develop recommendations that would lead to the solutions to the problems they identified as having national import. After the committee had completed an initial exploration of the problem, the foundation officers next asked a second task force of leaders in the ADN movement to advise them. They specifically asked for recommendations of ways the foundation could best support the continued growth of quality in the nation's more than 600 ADN programs.

The second task force agreed that assistance was needed to increase the number of adequately prepared faculty for ADN programs, to address the lack of consensus between nurse educators and nursing service personnel about entry-level competencies and differentiation of roles, and to explore the complaint of nursing service about the ADN graduate's weak clinical skills. The lack of a clear definition of the expected work role of the ADN graduate loomed large. What *was* the new graduate expected to do upon first coming to work?

A programming format for a project of national scope was agreed upon, and state and regional nursing organizations were invited to submit proposals for projects that would function as parts of the overall project and that would concern the preparation of the AD nurse and her use in hospitals upon graduation. The overall goal of all the projects was to improve nursing care by applying carefully taught theory to appropriate practice — that is, to end the separation of nursing education and nursing practice. A number of proposals were submitted. The foundation ultimately committed more than $6 million to fund six of them. All were based on the conviction that the resolution of differences between educators and hospital staff about the proper role of the AD nurse was essential to improving nursing practice in hospitals for all American citizens.

Regional and statewide organizations participated in the national effort: (1) the California statewide project, which was initiated by Ohlone College; (2) the Midwest Alliance in Nursing (MAIN); (3) the Southern Regional Education Board's (SREB) Southern Council on Collegiate Education for Nursing (SCCEN); and (4) the Western Interstate Council on

Higher Education's (WICHE) nursing council (WICHEN).

These projects were addressed to the basic and initial preparation of the AD nurse. The projects used various approaches, but all sites were concerned with determining the behaviors and knowledge to be expected from graduates of the different programs, with building consensus among nurse educators and hospital staffs, with determining learning experiences in the curricula for the various educational programs in nursing, and with building job descriptions and clinical ladder programs to demonstrate differences in the work role of the nurse.

In the sections that follow, each of these areas of concern—actually, steps taken toward the overall project goal—is described by using representative activities from the various individual projects. Specific activities have been selected to illustrate the variety of methods that the project participants used to achieve project goals. Although each subproject operated independently, subproject leaders met regularly to discuss problems and share insights. The overview of subproject work in this chapter attempts to show how the overall project, considered as a single entity, achieved results. The focus here is on the central goal of the national project.[4]

Reaching Consensus on the Work Role at Graduation

With the decline of the number of diploma programs, nurse educators and nursing practice directors and supervisors fell into an adversarial relationship. Practice personnel accused educators of failing to adequately prepare students for the realities of the work world. Educators countered that nursing service failed to use the AD graduate properly; they cited the lack of work role differentiation by level of preparation and the lack of job descriptions for various levels as evidence that nursing service had no understanding of the different levels of preparation for nursing. For its part, nursing service felt burdened by the need to provide extended orientation periods for ADN graduates, who often lacked the procedural skills they needed to practice successfully in hospitals. No small part of the burden was the cost, which grew to unprecedented levels.

Fundamentally, it was a policy question: Which was more important, easing the ADN graduate into her work role in the hospital setting as cost-effectively as possible or maintaining the initial purposes of the AD program? In the 1950s the founders of the ADN movement based the curriculum of the new program on the assumption that nursing tasks and knowledge varied along a continuum, from the simple to the complex. At the intermediate range was a set of functions they labeled "technical" and placed at the AD level in the educational system. The question that had yet to be answered concerned the actual work role of the graduate in hospitals. Does the graduate upon employment find that her employer's expectations for her performance exceed the middle range of abilities for which she has been prepared? And if the expectations do exceed the ability of the new graduate to perform, what can be done to correct the situation?

One prominent response to the problem was the numerous comprehensive lists of expected knowledge and behaviors of the novice nurse, expressed in the nursing literature as sets of competencies, which first appeared in the early 1970s. Initially embraced by ADN educators as the definitive means of proving the value of their programs and of defining their tier as different from that of other nurse education programs, such lists proliferated as many a faculty devoted considerable time and energy to working out its own version of the desired and expected competencies.

Competencies quickly became a hotly debated issue, as different groups had varied views of what the ADN and the BSN competencies should be. The debates among educators, hospital staffs, and students often degenerated into a power contest. Whose will was to prevail? Which lists were correct? And why were BSN competencies so much more difficult to address?

The sets of competencies multiplied. Regional nursing organizations, statewide planning groups, state boards of nursing, and individual programs and schools developed sets of competencies for their own use. In 1978 the NLN published what was purported to be the final word on the behaviors expected of the AD nurse upon graduation. In this list five broad areas were addressed: the nurse as a (1) provider of nursing care, (2) teacher, (3) communicator, (4) manager of care, and (5) member of the nursing community. Under each of these were arrayed the specific knowledge and behaviors to be considered by faculties constructing curricula.[5]

By the time the national Kellogg project was being assembled, nurses were so given to developing their own sets of competencies in preference to those of regional or national import that when WICHEN, one of the project's main subdivisions, set up its own projects, it expressly limited participants to three or four sets. No new competencies could be suggested by any group. Clearly, it was time to move on, to achieve consensus.

One concrete step toward defining the work role of the nurse in the hospital was taken when Ohlone College contracted with the California Board of Registered Nursing for a job analysis of all experienced and entry-level RNs working in the state. The purpose was to clearly define the functions, knowledge, and abilities that were critical to the safe and effective practice of entry-level nursing—and to do so on the basis of what was actually happening in nursing practice. The results of such an analysis would differ from the competency lists in a most important respect: they would be based on the facts of current practice rather than on a group's theoretical supposition about what should be happening in nursing practice.

The job analysis was subcontracted in part to Biddle and Associates, Inc., who supplied its own copyrighted methodology, Guidelines Oriented Job Analysis (GOJA), which had been used for more than ten years and had been approved in court as meeting federal job analysis and content validity standards. The subcontractor's method was to develop a comprehensive description of nursing practice on the basis of job content information obtained from a variety of knowledgeable sources. The functions, knowledge, and abilities identified were then fashioned into surveys to which nurses and other experts on the occupation could respond. Because there were so many job functions listed, four survey forms were written. Approximately 20,000 working nurses were asked to complete one of the four, and more than 4,000 did, resulting in a 22 percent response rate. Demographic information about the respondents was also collected. These responses were then used to verify the job content information that had been assembled initially. Further refinement was achieved by reviewing the literature on the content of nursing practice and by probing the job analysis in a series of intensive eight-hour workshops, in which nurses from throughout the state were asked to report what they actually did on the job and to identify the knowledge and abilities that were required.

Job analysis standards require that objective data be collected on how often functions are performed, on the importance of a poor performance on nursing care, and on the connection of knowledge and abilities to actual job functions. The analysis that the subcontractor supplied was an exhaustive listing of the content of RN practice that specified nursing function, applied knowledge and abilities, tools and equipment used by RNs, physical requirements, employment terms and conditions, and contact with other employers. An initial list of 2,000 items was honed to a final list of 598 functions and 360 knowledges and abilities.

In addition to identifying job functions, the subcontractor analyzed the demographic information to distinguish the entry-level skills from those of the experienced nurses. The threshold between the two levels was defined as occurring at the point at which a nurse indicates her ability to perform a function without guidance. The subcontractor determined that this threshold is usually crossed by a nurse after seventeen months of practice, depending somewhat on previous experience and other variables. It was also determined that experienced nurses tend to perform a larger number of functions than do novice nurses. The difference, the facts indicated, is attributable to the fact that entry-level nurses are not needed to perform certain functions, not that they are unable to perform them.

A most important finding of this review of the specific job functions in hospital nursing indicated a high focus on clinical judgment and decision making in nursing practice. No longer could there be any doubt that the cognitive aspects of practice are what separate the RN from all nursing assistant positions. The project also provided the empirical evidence that defines nursing as a complex endeavor requiring a large number of various skills and knowledge that are difficult to cover in a short education program—a fact known intuitively by nurses but largely unrecognized by the public. The subcontractor, who based his estimate of the fee for the job on the basis of his experience performing such job analyses for other health care occupations, seriously underbid the contract. It turned out that the nursing role, regardless of level of educational preparation, is far more complex than had been generally assumed.

The California study did not differentiate the roles of nurses prepared at the associate degree and the baccalaureate levels, but it certainly can be concluded from the study that hospital practice demands much more than is implied by the stereotypical image of the nurse simply as a hands-on performer. Publication of the study should enhance the public image of the nurse as a knowledgeable practitioner of a highly developed discipline.

The primary intent of other work done in California was to test the validity of the list of competencies developed by the NLN and to demonstrate that they work. Project participants developed ways to measure the behavior in question, inserted the opportunity to learn the precursor behaviors in the curriculum or learning environment, and empirically tested the learner and the learning experience for the resultant behavior.

Altogether, the California projects attempted to answer three basic questions that had troubled the nursing community for some time:

1. What can the ADN graduate do immediately upon graduation?
2. What can the graduate do six months later?
3. What does the employer expect the graduate to do at these times?

The results exceeded expectations. The most important conclusions drawn from several different parts of the project were these:

1. ADN graduating students, their faculty, older graduates, and their supervisors rated the clinical performance of the average AD nurse as satisfactory or better on all five role dimensions identified by the NLN—teacher, communicator, care provider, care manager, and member of the profession.
2. The percentage of ADN graduates rating their own performance as satisfactory or better ranged from a low of 83 percent for client teacher to a high of 99 percent for patient communicator.
3. Supervisors rated 84 percent of ADN graduates as satisfactory or better in all five roles.
4. Most supervisors (84 to 91 percent) reported critical care skills and managerial abilities as being either important or essential for a beginning staff nurse.
5. ADN graduates rated their own education preparation as satisfactory or better for all five roles.

Although critical care skills had not been included in the usual repertoire of abilities expected of the ADN graduate, nor had managerial skills beyond those used in the care of the individual patient, many projects in the overall Kellogg effort revealed the rapprochement that had been reached since 1979 between nursing service administrators and nurse educators about the work role of the AD nurse. Whether nursing educators were doing a better job or practice personnel were finally adjusting their expectations to the work role as taught by AD faculties was unanswered.

In some project locations across the nation, participants discovered to their surprise that the level of agreement between nursing service and education was much higher than they had expected. It seemed that the problem had not been dissimilar goals, as most had believed, but, rather, lack of communication. What nurse educators and nursing practice administrators were finding was that, although the two groups might not use the same words to describe their objectives, their ideas were the same. Reaching agreement about entry-level competencies turned out to be the easiest part of the project task.

Indeed, some states had reached agreement on competencies; for example, Arizona had its "Inventory of Competencies and Skills for ADN Graduates," which had been approved by the Arizona State Board of Community Colleges in 1979. Mississippi also had a listing of expected competencies approved by the state's educational governing bodies. South Carolina's Statewide Master Planning Committee had determined ADN and BSN competencies for its own use, and the SNAP project in New Mexico had determined competencies for that state. The competencies developed in the SREB's curriculum project were widely accepted in the South. In some instances competencies were determined by ad hoc committees. However, in other localities, work on competencies continued, and consensus was yet to be fully achieved. Consultants were brought to various sites to assist teams with consensus building; NLN competencies were modified; and an opinion survey was conducted in Hawaii.

Nurses in the Midwest portion of the project conducted a literature search for the definitions of nursing, nursing role and how it is defined, differentiated levels of practice, and role statements prepared by others. They also reviewed terminal objectives of various kinds of nurse education programs, identified enabling behaviors to reach the objectives, and specified evaluation criteria to ensure that the objectives had been met.

The work on the enabling behaviors took an enormous amount of time. Pairs of observers from practice and education went into hospital units to observe nurses in practice for two-hour periods. The total number of observational hours was quite large. All shifts were covered, as behaviors were found to be shift related. From this large database the project developed job descriptions, tools for evaluating job performance, and an orientation guide to differentiated practice.

The communication networks created during project work were

one of its most positive results. In the South, for example, the project established model demonstration sites at six ADN programs that, being open to all interested persons, served as a means for improving the communication between nurse educators and service administrators. Retreat teams in projects throughout the country came to know and respect one another. New working relationships were established. Indeed, a new climate for working together was created. Knowledge was shared and misconceptions erased, and people gained insight into the constraints that others worked under.

Methods of reaching consensus by local mutual agreement were a strength of projects across the nation. Even more strength would come from agreed-upon national goals for the work role of the ADN and the BSN nurse in the hospital. If AD nursing exemplifies one nursing role, an intermediate set of functions, can it be teased apart from the professional one? Could a team of educators and practitioners readily agree upon the professional role? Questions such as these remained unanswered.

WICHEN at the beginning of its project called both the ANA and the NLN to ask for samples of just such differentiated practice in hospitals. Neither organization could refer the WICHEN staff to a single site that could provide the samples sought. Yet, to define the ADN role without a similar definition of the other, the BSN, role seemed foolhardy.

"It is highly regrettable," Montag had said, "that the planned development of baccalaureate programs did not take place simultaneously with the associate degree." Instead, "associate degree programs had to contend with the popular view that all nurses are alike. The belief I held at that time [1952, when the earliest programs were being established under the CRP]—and still do—was that diploma programs prepared technicians (and not very well at that) and that few baccalaureate programs were, in fact, providing professional education." In sum, in Montag's view, ADN graduates were being prepared for a new role, but no complementary role was being created for the baccalaureate graduate.[6] The view is quite controversial, and not many nurse educators would agree, but the lack of communication among nurse educators is quite evident in such a statement.

In May of 1983 WICHEN asked the Kellogg Foundation for additional funding of an exploratory study of the similarities and differences between the technical and professional role. A task force of educators and executive-level nursing administrators was asked to reach consensus on BSN competencies, to ascertain whether graduates were actually prepared to assume the role and to evaluate the extent to which nursing service expects and provides novices the opportunity to practice that role.

As with the work done in defining the ADN role, the task force was restricted to competing statements already developed by the ANA (1981), the NLN (1983), New Mexico (SNAP, 1979), and the Orange County Consortium (1981). After the work role for both the AD and the BSN nurses had been defined in terms of competencies and the lists mailed to all the schools in the West, a survey form listing each competency was mailed to hospitals and other community health agencies:

1. Do you expect the graduate to perform or possess this skill or ability?
2. Do they have an opportunity in your setting to practice this skill or employ this ability?
3. Do the graduates come to your agency able to perform this competency?

The detailed results of this study have been published and are readily available.[7] It is important for our purposes to note that the BSN graduate was rated as satisfactory immediately upon graduation in seven of ten categories that defined the expected role for a provider of care. The BSN graduate rates a satisfactory label in the other three competencies at the end of the second year of employment. Similar results were reported for performance in all other areas—communicator, teacher, investigator and member of the nursing discipline, planner and organizer—with the exception of the role of investigator, referring to the nurses' research abilities. The results of the rating of the ADN graduates were essentially the same. On many more competencies the novice graduates performed they were rated as unprepared to practice upon initial employment, but all performances, with the exception of the role as investigator, were satisfactory by the end of the second year.

Other sites across the country used different means of arriving at the BSN work role as distinguished from the ADN role, but all who worked on the problem found that an understanding of both was essential to the building of curricula and the establishment of job descriptions and clinical ladders—the next tasks of the project.

Effecting Change after Consensus

Once consensus on the work roles—defined as differing competencies —had been reached, the project participants could turn to the task of bringing the ADN curricula at project sites across the country in line with the new agreements. Methods for doing this differed but generally included (1) changing the curriculum, (2) revising the expectations of clinical performance, and (3) planning for the transition from student to working nurse.

Changing the Curriculum

Curricular changes were directed toward revising the educational objectives for each year's content, writing modular instructional packages, and developing clinical content to reflect the actual practice situation. The enhancement of clinical performance centered on skills lists. The project leaders focused on improving assessment skills and decision-making abilities; they revised clinical evaluation tools and improved clinical competency examinations. They planned for the transition from student to nurse by developing new hospital orientation programs and using preceptors during the last year of the nursing education program. Both proved helpful in orienting the novice to the work setting.

For example, SREB demonstration centers established by the project each focused on a specific theme, many having substantial implications for curricular change. One center concentrated on curriculum construction, another on the development of instructional packages, and still another on competency-based planning for the student's transition to the work role.

Revising Expectations of Clinical Performance. It was easier to determine the employer's expectations of the new graduate's knowledge and behavior than to assure the employer that the novice had mastered and could perform a particular competency. In both the surveys conducted in the West, educators had ranked their graduates as being more capable than their service counterparts had ranked them. These results demonstrated clearly to educators that they needed a better system of evaluating clinical competency if they were to be able to incorporate appropriate teaching methods into the curriculum. Moreover, service people needed a reliable system of evaluation in order to assess job performance. Unless the identified competencies were measurable and were reflected in actual performance, they would have little meaning.

To address these issues, one project conducted a series of faculty staff development activities to increase everyone's skill in evaluating clinical competencies. Self-evaluation methods and regional workshops were used to identify the primary needs of faculty and hospital staff. The most difficult areas in evaluating clinical competence were (1) limited time, (2) lack of clear identification of the behaviors to be evaluated, and (3) lack of guidelines for evaluating high-level cognitive abilities.

The project then developed a program, "Objective Assessment of Clinical Competence," composed of a manual and an interactive video-conference. The manual taught the basic concepts of clinical evaluation and allowed each participant to conduct a self-assessment of practice and knowledge. The video-conference was viewed at ten sites throughout the state in October 1983 and was attended by 330 nurses, two-thirds of whom were educators and the other third, service personnel. Regional workshops to reinforce knowledge and skills followed. Options were offered for those unable to attend scheduled workshops, including the viewing of the October videotaped conference, completing the manual, and attending subregional workshops.

Bringing about specific changes in the work environment was a most important result of the joint planning by educators and service administrators. One of the purposes of the overall project was to address the complaint of nursing service that the ADN graduate's clinical skills were weak upon initial employment. Upon finding that their complaint was the consequence of a misunderstanding of what the ADN graduate could be expected to do upon initial employment, nursing service people began to experiment with changes in some of their procedures. For example, the Arizona project revised job descriptions and other personnel practices, including the preparation of clinical evaluation tools for clinical placement; Colorado established joint appointments to plan for better use of staff nurse competencies; Idaho devised performance evaluation tools to be used three, six, and twelve months after graduation; New Mexico established a transitional mentor program; a program in the state of Washington created clinical ladder programs based on competency-based evaluation tools for staff nurses and novices; and many locations at other project sites developed new job descriptions based on the competency consensus determined earlier.

For example, the Rideout Hospital-Yuba team developed a job analysis instrument based on NLN competencies and put into a nursing process format. Sixty-six members of a special task force made up, reviewed, revised, and rank-ordered each item of the tool. Forty job descriptions were collected, and graduates and supervisors were surveyed about entry-level nursing tasks. Analysis of the data culminated in a "realistic, behaviorally oriented, entry-level job description and performance evaluation tool" for local use at several institutions. The tool is used for ADN students prior to graduation and again six months after their entry into practice. "Holding new graduates accountable for retraining and using the knowledge and skills deemed critical by both service and education," the project reported, "increases [the] cost effectiveness of orientation and in-service programs by reducing the time required and narrowing the scope of hospital-specific requirements." The job description is designed for several uses: in a hospital orientation program, for appraisal of performance by staff and by students themselves, and as a guideline for professional development by all nurses. This newly developed tool is now in use at both Rideout Hospital and Yuba College.

The educators at Yuba were surprised that they could so easily work with in-service educators and other nursing service personnel. They discovered that their expectations of nursing performance were alike, that their goals were the same, and, ultimately, that working together was profoundly satisfying. Their next task was to assemble a clinical ladder based on their mutually agreed-upon expectations. They matched curricular content with job expectations and on this basis created a model for continuing consultation and collaboration between the academic and the practice settings. As a consequence, the students' expectations gained in school matched their initial experience at work. The good fit was the direct result of the successful establishment of local performance behaviors.

Planning for Transition from Novice Status. Many sites in the national project addressed aspects of the problems of the novice, developing and testing ways to make the transition smoother and less costly for all concerned.

As an example, Solano Community College began by validating the NLN competency statements relating to the role of manager of care for the individual client. Initially, a joint service-education committee was formed to select the behaviors that would demonstrate a novice's attainment of competency in this role. Critical behaviors were identified for each competency listed for the role. The behaviors were then used to plan a preceptorship program in leadership, which included a specially designed learning module and a competency-based examination of performance.

The collection of data to help faculty measure leadership outcomes began in 1983–1984. The Schwirian six-dimension scale of nursing performance and the Managerial Key of the California Psychological Inventory (CPI) were selected for use in a pretest-posttest design to measure the effectiveness of the preceptorship program. Six months after graduation Solano students scored higher on their student pretest scores on the Schwirian instrument but showed no change on the managerial key. Preceptors were asked to rate their preceptees on the twenty nursing behaviors listed by the NLN for the nurse-manager role. At the end of the four-week period, they rated students as being able to perform nineteen of the twenty functions by the time of graduation. Self-evaluation of performance proved to be the only troublesome category among the twenty.

Generally, all concerned considered the preceptorship a success. Staff nurse preceptors evaluated students as being more capable than they had expected they would rate them. The students reported an increased self-confidence and independence, plus a better ability to organize and set priorities in patient care. Their perception of their work roles as nurses was changed, becoming more realistic.

Faculty at Solano College plan to continue the service-education committee and annually to evaluate the nursing curriculum, the preceptorship program, and the performance examination to measure managerial role behaviors. Having found a means to solve a sore problem, these project participants have elected to refine it and keep putting it to work.

Building Differentiated Work Roles

All subdivisions of the national project deliberated at length the issue of differentiation, and all found that consensus on the different work roles of the BSN and the ADN graduates was easily reached. One of the projects took the process one step further, mounting an effort to demonstrate the workability of the differentiated roles.

After reaching consensus on the work role of the staff nurse, midwestern nurses participating in the project determined upon a clinical trial to test their set of differentiated competencies, or, as some called them, terminal objectives. Hospital units for demonstrating differentiated practice were selected at three sites: Harper, Grace, and Hatzell hospitals in Michigan.

In the first phase of the effort, BSN-prepared head nurses were asked to volunteer to participate in the establishment of the unit. The usual staffing patterns continued during this phase, but each head nurse was oriented to the different roles of the ADN and the BSN graduates, as outlined by the midwestern project members and translated into protocols describing the expected role of each staff member. Job descriptions were used that had been tested and correlated with the competencies developed by the project.

The second stage of the process involved the actual assignments to care dictated by the project assumptions about the work roles of the ADN and the BSN nurse. Using primary nursing as the assignment method of choice, the project assigned the role as case manager to BSN graduates and the role as case associate to AD and diploma nurses. The difference in role was sometimes demonstrated to head nurses by faculty participation. A checklist of skills and a proficiency measurement tool had been developed for both roles, and staff member participants were asked to complete the tool at the end of each day's work. Audits to confirm the proper assignments were a part of the process of evaluating the efficacy of the unit. In addition, unit observations were made by knowledgeable observers, and preceptors working with novice staff members kept diaries.

The differentiated unit established by the project at Harper Hospital, thought to be the first in the nation, was highly successful. Since that time, units have been put in place by the Yale New Haven Hospital and the Sioux Valley Hospital in South Dakota; perhaps others, unknown to us at this writing, have been established as well.

Conclusions

As the projects completed their work, it became apparent that a consensus had been reached by nursing service and nursing education about the entry-level work role of the AD nurse—no mean achievement. Great strides had been made in defining and putting into place differentiated practice roles. Such differentiation made it possible for each novice nurse to be used in the hospital in the role for which she had been educated and prepared. Troublesome issues associated with the novice's adjustment to the work setting could now be put aside.

Both service and education gained new insights in working through the project task. "I didn't know they did that," expressed with frank surprise, was a constant refrain. In every state many people admitted to their astonishment that all could agree and work together so effectively. Their surprise on both counts testifies to the seriousness of the rift that had developed over the years. In working together, project participants from service and education had learned that their expectations were apparently similar, though the words they used to describe them had been different.

The complaint about the ADN graduates' weak clinical skills disappeared in the light of the facts. Knowledge about the community college preparatory program assured nurses working in hospitals that the AD nurse was receiving proper instruction. To enhance the clinical portion of the curriculum, educators separated their clinical teaching methods from their clinical evaluation methods, teaching at one specific time, evaluating at another. They targeted exact behaviors for measurement rather than broadly defined abilities and thought processes. Competency-based testing, targeted to specific goals, was developed and used successfully. Curricular offerings, when found wanting, were revised to bring them in line with the realities of the workplace. Preceptorships coupling the student or the novice with an experienced nurse for the purpose of teaching specific clinical abilities were widely used in the project and were judged useful by many nurses across the country.

The usual novice period for the AD nurse in hospitals was defined empirically by the project. In the California Board of Registered Nursing study the period was determined to be seventeen months, and in the WICHEN studies, two years. The novice who would be oriented to hospital policies and procedures immediately upon graduation was now a figure of the past, as even the hospital-based programs that remain today are more pedagogically structured than formerly. The costs of the novice period are a permanent part of the budget for hospital nursing services.

The nation's first differentiated practice unit was established by the project in Michigan. Job descriptions based upon an agreed-upon work role for the AD nurse were put in place, clinical ladders for promotion based on an individual nurse's expanded performance and knowledge base were considered, and novice program planning resulted from the cooperative efforts of nurse educators and their nursing practice counterparts.

Nurses working in the various subprojects found that working together was addicting; most simply wanted more. Joint education-service groups that were disbanded after the project work had been completed asked to continue meeting. The members were willing to commute long distances, if necessary, to gain the benefits of exchanging ideas and discussing mutual concerns.

Offshoots from the central task were commonplace at many sites. Faculty and nursing practice personnel exchanged teaching responsibilities. Hospital staff taught classes at the college, and faculty offered continuing education courses at the hospital. Joint marketing and recruiting campaigns were also mounted. One preceptorship program was the subject of a hospital's advertisements for staff. Hospital equipment was on occasion donated to the colleges. In one instance the cooperative relationship resulted in the hospital's operating as defender of the ADN program; when an educational program review of the nursing program recommended a cutback in enrollments, the local hospital pressed for reconsideration, and the recommendation for the cutback was withdrawn.

Lasting relationships were established by continued committee exchanges, monthly meetings, and in a few instances a joint appointment of faculty and hospital staff to the same institution. In California the goal of establishing a basis for ongoing communication between education and service was better realized than project planners had expected. Although the California statewide project ended in 1985, the collaborative efforts between service and education have continued. The evaluation method developed by a joint committee in the project now is being used as the model for a job evaluation tool being developed by several hospitals in Santa Barbara. Likewise, the SREB demonstration sites created new avenues of communication that participants were determined to continue to use, informally as well as formally, wherever possible.

Finally, it can be said that nursing service representatives participating in the project who were appointed to joint committees learned firsthand what the ADN program's didactic and clinical experiences contained. As a result, they knew better what to expect of the ADN graduate in the workplace. The hospitals were now able to match their expectations to the realities of ADN education and thus to improve their employment practices. In the WICHEN project, for example, administrators in rural hospitals and long-term care facilities found that they required the BSN graduate.

With the work role of the ADN graduate now clearly defined, surprises for both the nurse and the hospital upon the nurse's initial employment could be eliminated. A practice niche for the ADN had at long last been clearly established.

ADN Faculty Preparation

In the early 1960s the NLN began to study the leading problems confronting ADN programs, which between 1960 and 1963 nearly doubled in number, from 57 to 105 programs.[1] Rapid growth was itself a problem. In January 1962 the NLN board approved a joint statement by the NLN and the AAJC that detailed the urgent need for faculty to serve as instructors and administrators in the newly developing ADN programs. The two organizations agreed to encourage senior colleges and universities to direct resources toward the development of baccalaureate nursing programs. Their reasoning was that these programs, by providing the basic collegiate education of nurses, formed the foundation of the graduate education of recruits for ADN teaching and administration.

Government officials, from the federal level on down, were uncomfortably aware of the shortage of ADN educators. In 1965 the surgeon general of the United States predicted a 44.5 percent increase in ADN graduates by 1970. Approximately 250 junior and community colleges had expressed an interest in developing ADN programs; these programs would require at least 2,000 new staff members. It was not just the nursing program that was developing so rapidly; junior colleges generally were experiencing explosive growth: 30 to 35 new colleges a year were opening their doors, and by 1964 junior and community college students accounted for nearly a fifth of the total postsecondary enrollment in the country.[2]

In 1964 Thomas B. Merton surveyed junior college presidents to ask them to describe the methods they were using to recruit nursing faculty and to suggest ways to increase the number of nurse faculty available for employment. The replies Merton received almost unanimously suggested that a nationwide effort was needed to establish graduate programs to train new nursing instructors throughout the nation in carefully selected universities. At the time only three universities offered special programs to prepare ADN faculty: Teachers College at Columbia University, UCLA, and the University of Florida.[3] Obviously, such numbers were far too low.

In 1965 the W. K. Kellogg Foundation, in response to the Merton survey, granted the AAJC funds to plan and conduct a conference for the purpose of assisting universities to design faculty training programs for ADN schools. The Conference on the Preparation of Instructors and Directors of ADN Programs was held at O'Hare Inn, Chicago, in April 1965. The conference focused attention first on the kinds of programs that would be needed, both in the short and the long term, and on the resources that would be required. It identified the jumping-off position most of those attending considered the most effective place to start: a joint NLN-AAJC Nursing Committee. Upon returning home each nursing dean who had attended prepared a statement of resources needed to extend efforts in teacher preparation in her state.[4]

In fact, between 1965 and 1968 the W. K. Kellogg Foundation embarked on the next step of a master plan to support associate degree education for nurses by focusing on the preparation of faculty specifically to teach in ADN programs. Several universities instituted projects to plan for curricular modification of the teacher-preparation portions of their offerings, to prepare nurses for beginning teaching positions in junior colleges, and to provide consultation services to developing ADN programs within their regional service areas.

In 1966 the foundation awarded Boston University a grant in support of its development of a master's program to prepare ADN faculty for junior colleges. It also awarded funds for similar programs at the University of Washington, Wayne State University, and the University of California at San Francisco. In 1967 Kellogg granted the University of Kentucky funds to develop a program at the master's level to prepare ADN teachers. Up to that time there had never been a master's nursing program in the state, which between 1963 and 1967 had greatly increased its commitment to AD nursing, in terms of both financial support and number of programs. In the face of such expansion at the junior college level, the state desperately needed qualified faculty.[5]

Indeed, the needs throughout the nation were so acute that graduate programs with strict residency requirements could not meet the needs of most states. Only the short-term continuing education courses being offered by scattered junior colleges and universities seemed to fill that gap. In 1965 the Kellogg Foundation renewed its support of the short-term program at Manatee Junior College in Florida, a state where community and junior colleges had been particularly numerous and successful. Manatee had previously served as a demonstration site for the four-state project. During the 1965–1966 academic year, for example, fifty-three faculty members from ADN programs throughout the nation visited the demonstration center. In 1966–1967 the site drew sixty-six visiting faculty; in 1967–1968, ninety-seven; and in 1968–1969, seventy-three. The visitors were provided with either a one-week intensive session or a three-week course, at the end of which they would elect one of two methods for follow-up, a site visit to their own institution by Manatee staff or an alternative plan of their own design.[6]

Also in 1965 the foundation funded a workshop intended to assist faculties in Michigan's junior colleges to improve their curricula for ADN programs. The workshop, held at Henry Ford Community College in June 1965, was led by Ruth Matheney, of Nassau Community College in New York.[7] The following year, in July, the foundation funded a workshop held under the auspices of the Southern Regional Education Board at the University of Tennessee at Memphis. This seminar resulted in a useful publication on the ADN curriculum that included a film list and a bibliography. During the same month another Kellogg-funded workshop on associate degree education was held at the University of Colorado. Mildred Montag served as the resource person for this occasion.[8] In 1967, this time in June, the foundation sponsored yet another seminar on ADN education at the University of Tennessee at Memphis. At nearly the same time a summer workshop on AD nursing was held at New York University, the Division of Nurse Education, with cooperating faculty from the ADN programs at Bronx Community College and Manatee Junior College in Florida.[9]

By 1970 the foundation was receiving reports from the master's programs to which it had awarded funds; these reports contain important information about the ways that master's-level preparation of ADN education was evolving. Wayne State reported that it had been able to meet its goals: it had reorganized an existing master's in nursing program to meet the specific needs of people who were already working in ADN programs but who lacked preparation in teaching. In so doing it had modified its curriculum, recruited additional faculty, and mounted cooperative programs with other institutions to provide more continuing education. Wayne State had tried a summers-only program but without success, because enrollment was low.[10]

The Boston University program reported that it had developed a two-semester, six-credit-hour course concerned with curricular development and teaching, which provided field experience in ADN teaching. Students were encouraged to adapt the course to meet their own needs as ADN educators. In addition, the university planned and conducted a series of conferences targeted to the needs of ADN faculty throughout New England. A motivational conference taught by Harvard University psychologists attracted twenty ADN faculty members from throughout the region. A two-day conference on creativity drew thirty-five; it was planned and conducted by faculty from Boston University, Boston College, and Harvard. In addition, consultation with university personnel was offered to institutions planning to open new ADN programs, and a faculty consultation conference led by twelve experts in ADN education was attended by more than one hundred ADN instructors. Summer work conferences on the preparation of ADN faculty were attended by seventy-five people. The project had succeeded in reaching well beyond the city of Boston to assist in ADN development throughout the New England area.[11] A clearinghouse for technical nursing literature and a placement service for ADN programs seeking faculty were established.

The project based at the University of Washington and directed by Doris Geitgey reported that it had adapted existing master's level courses in nursing research, practice teaching, and independent study to focus on the preparation of ADN faculty. Moreover, university faculty members provided consultation services and offered summer workshops for ADN educators. The goals of the project were to (1) recruit and prepare master's students for leadership and teaching positions in ADN programs, (2) develop a sequence of seminars beyond the master's level on ADN education, (3) provide summer workshops for ADN faculty, and (4) introduce students to part-time work-study programs in ADN nursing. The project surveyed each master's class regarding students' career goals and learned that it was succeeding in increasing the number of students who were planning to enter ADN education.[12]

New York University sought to assist diploma faculty to prepare for teaching in the ADN program. The NYU graduate faculty were also interested in preparing faculty to work in inner-city programs. The University of California at Berkeley offered workshops and other continuing education programs for faculty and others interested in the sound development of technical nursing education.[13]

The number of special and continuing education programs could not keep pace with the demand for ADN teachers, despite the best efforts of the many sponsoring schools and the support of the foundations, most notably of course the Kellogg Foundation. Federal assistance proved to be essential to providing the number of people needed to fill faculty positions.

Many new ADN faculty members were prepared for junior college teaching with the assistance of federal traineeship funds. By 1972 more than 63,000 nurses had received federal awards, but even this number had not been enough to meet the demand for teachers. By 1982, just ten years later, the situation was little improved. An estimate of the number of instructors teaching in ADN programs without holding a master's degree in nursing showed regional variation, but nonetheless few states met the recommended standard. States moving in that direction were governed by state boards of nursing that required the master's in nursing as a credential for teaching.

Kellogg's Renewed Initiative to Prepare ADN Faculty

The foundation's ad hoc advisory committee on ADN education, meeting in the late 1970s, again recommended attention to the preparation of faculty for the ADN program. As a part of the third step of the master plan to assist AD nursing, the Kellogg Foundation selected six sites across the country in 1982 to serve as demonstration areas for establishing a master's degree in nursing especially geared to preparing faculty for ADN programs. In the West, the University of Portland, a private university serving Oregon and close-by western states, and the University of California, with its "1,000-mile campus" and a main office in Long Beach, provided project sites. In the South, the University of South Florida in Tampa and the University of Tennessee in Knoxville were participants. In the Midwest, the University of Nebraska in Omaha and the University of Oklahoma's Health Science Center in Oklahoma City agreed to participate.[14]

Initial assessment of need for the graduate program at individual sites was representative of the national picture. In Tennessee, for example, the nursing faculty surveyed the sixteen ADN programs in the state. Of the 196 nursing faculty employed by these programs, only 106 held the MSN degree, fifty-five held the BSN as the highest credential, and two held neither the master's nor the bachelor's degree. Five of the ADN programs were new and had not hired their full complement of faculty at the time of the survey.

Only twenty-six of the 140 nursing faculty employed in diploma programs in the state held the MSN degree. The majority of these programs were engaged in phase-out planning, and their faculty members would not be qualified to obtain positions in ADN or BSN programs without additional preparation. Family responsibilities and lack of access to graduate education in nursing had caused several to obtain master's degrees in other fields, usually education, and three of the students held doctorates in education. Some of the students reported that the only person in their nursing program holding a graduate degree in nursing was their director. During the initial phase of the project the director recalled interviewing a prospective student who headed an ADN program in North Carolina; neither the director nor any of her faculty held a master's degree in nursing.

In Florida an initial needs assessment indicated that approximately 50 percent of those persons currently teaching in ADN programs did not hold the MSN degree. Because of a lack of access to nursing master's programs offered at a time acceptable to the working student, there was a backlog of students who wanted to enroll in a flexible program. As a consequence, at least two teachers with twenty-five years' experience entered and graduated from the program. A few other teachers held master's and doctoral degrees, particularly in education, but not the master's degree in nursing required by accrediting bodies for teaching in the ADN program.

Clearly, a graduate program was much needed at each site, one that could provide the appropriate educational content for nurses teaching or aspiring to teach in the ADN program and one that could also offer nontraditional programming that would be accessible to working nurse educators who could not leave their jobs to attend graduate school.

Each master's program in the project was asked to adapt its curriculum to the student preparing for a teaching career in basic nursing education at the AD level. Programs were also to offer clinical preparation in two practice areas, as the ADN curriculum required teachers working in a broad-fields curriculum to teach more than one specialty practice area to basic students. Adherents of AD nursing were strongly in favor of this practice, but, as it turned out, graduate faculty and students were less supportive of the notion.

The effort at the six sites touched thousands of American lives. Individuals teaching in ADN programs or aspiring to do so benefited financially and educationally. A teacher with twenty-five years' experience returned to school. A father and daughter enrolled as master's students at the Tampa site. Persons with master's and doctoral degrees in other disciplines returned to nursing colleges to prepare for ADN teaching roles. Women with more than two children also in college were students at Portland. Faculty working in programs where no teacher was educationally prepared for her job enrolled in the Tennessee program. More than four hundred students signed up for the nontraditional master's program in California, many of them already ADN faculty members. A student in the Oklahoma program traveled more than a thousand miles from her home each week to attend master's classes.

The Student Need for Access

One of the most important contributions this group of projects made to increasing the number of new ADN teachers was in providing access to master's programs at times and places that working women with family responsibilities could manage. Students attended not only because of the desire for a teaching credential but also because a master's degree was attainable in a schedule that fit their lifestyle.

Students evaluating the California program, who were typical of students in all the others, were enthusiastic about its accessibility. Responses to questions posed to students about the strengths of the program included these: "flexible hours for classes especially on weekends and evenings," "proximity of classes to my home," "flexibility of course work," "offers classes for the working nurse," "it allows a person to work full time and attend," "convenience," and "it facilitates advanced education for those who cannot move and attend a full-time program."

Overwhelmingly, students in all six programs were part-time learners (68 percent) who worked from thirty-one to forty hours each week (65 percent). It would have been unrealistic to expect them to fit traditional graduate study into their busy lives. Rigid residency requirements were impossible for them to meet. When students from throughout the nation were queried about their reasons for enrolling in the master's program, 83 percent cited the location of the program and 48 percent cited the program's flexibility as the reasons for enrolling. The features the students liked most about their master's programs were the self-paced learning (49 percent), classes with seminar format (41 percent), and the location of classes off campus (35 percent).

Access to didactic and clinical coursework that fits within the existing framework of a student's life therefore became the most important ingredient for success. Students participating in the project were assured that they could complete the degree requirements because their access to all program elements was carefully protected. The California program is especially useful to illustrate the strategies for accomplishing this.

The California program required no on-campus theoretical or clinical coursework. Courses were delivered through independent study modules and intensive weekend seminars held in regional satellite locations. The mission of the "1,000-mile campus" program was, in the view of the faculty, on the cutting edge of the nontraditional programs in nursing. The baccalaureate program had ninety-six sites in eighteen regions in California, enrolling about 4,000 students. The master's program was located in five regional sites, none of which had a traditional master's program. The enrollment was 455 students, of which 153 had elected to prepare for teaching in the ADN program. All sites were in the southern part of the state, with the exception of San Luis Obispo, which is centrally located. Reluctance to establish service agreements had been encountered by some institutions, but generally the acceptance of the nontraditional programs had been good, especially by students.

Students were recruited by way of statewide mailing lists and word of mouth in nursing circles. The cost of the program to both institution and student was higher than traditional master's programs, but the students' tuition and fees plus grants that faculty were able to attract made the program self-supporting. The possibility of bringing the program under the formula-based funding mechanism used for traditional programs in the state is now under consideration.

One key to the success of the nontraditional California program was the careful focus on and monitoring of student life. Before taking their first course, students registered for a workshop that faculty viewed as an advanced orientation program. It was held at numerous hospitals and medical centers throughout the state. At these workshops students were led through the learning strategies and expectations for (1) successful performance, (2) program planning, (3) writing and speaking requirements, and (4) resource identification in the student's place of residence. It was determined whether a student had access to MEDLINE and three libraries containing a health care collection. Students' computer literacy was assessed. The workshops also addressed strategies for academic success in self-directed learning, writing skills, learning word processing, traditional library research skills, gaining the encouragement of friends and peers, carpooling, and sharing residences for weekend seminars. Moreover, students were eased into the program: they began their graduate work by taking only one unit of a nursing theory course, in part to allow themselves time to make lifestyle adjustments before accelerating the academic pace.

Learning resource centers containing print materials and learning technology hardware and software were established in a variety of educational and health care institutions, and students were provided library privileges at the branches of the University of California and California State University libraries in their local communities.

After admission to the nursing program and upon enrollment in a first course, the student received books and materials via UPS. Course modules provided detailed learning plans, evaluation criteria, and several photocopied journal articles that were part of a required reading list. Videotapes housed in the satellite learning centers were adjuncts to the module content in some instances. The student engaged in considerable preparation before the first seminar of the course was held and then was guided by a learning packet for continued preparation for other, more advanced lessons. Seminars were devoted to discussion and informed debate about the learning material. By preparing oral presentations and scholarly papers, students could demonstrate their newly acquired knowledge.

The modules developed at the California site are self-contained learning packages resembling the highly acclaimed modules developed for the undergraduate program. Consultants who were experts in their respective nursing disciplines were used to prepare the materials for the master's program. After course outlines were prepared, texts examined, and syllabi developed, faculty members reviewed the materials and suggested revisions. Each module was reviewed by six faculty members as well as the program director and the curriculum coordinator. Later revisions were based on evaluations of students and instructors, or designed to reflect advances in nursing knowledge. Instructors at the eleven satellite sites were permitted to elaborate on the content of modules but not to eliminate assignments or make substantial changes. Standardization of the courses across the state was thus protected.

Once accepted into the program and having paid a program fee, each student was appointed a mentor. The mentor was more than an advisor in the traditional sense; each mentor was expected to establish close personal relationships with her students, to serve as a role model, and to perform the traditional duties of an advisor: planning programs of study and assisting students with academic problems. Students and mentors were matched on the basis of geographic location and the functional role the students had chosen to study (teacher, administrator, or clinical specialist). Mentors attended the orientation program and frequently served as instructors. After completing orientation, students proceeded through the course of master's study, usually taking two to three years to complete the program.

The nontraditional educational practices described for California were also in place at the other project sites across the country. In the interest of telling the story without redundancy, we are emphasizing only the variations from the standard pattern that made each site unique.

Students were attracted to the program in Oregon because it could be completed in three summers, with nine credits earned elsewhere, or in two summers, using specially developed nontraditional courses. Here, too, the fact that a program could be made to fit around the other demands of a busy adult's life was a key element in its success.

The Portland site attracted students from a number of western states besides Oregon—Washington, North Dakota, Montana, and Alaska. But it was not unusual for students from as far away as New York, Florida, or Arizona to enroll. International students were also attracted—from Kuwait, Japan, British Columbia and other Canadian provinces.

The university initially supported a local hospital-based program but soon developed its own BSN program and in 1977 pioneered with a summer-only master's program. Faculty report that the summer is the busiest and in many respects the most rewarding time in the work year.

Students at the University of South Florida (USF) could do clinical practicums wherever they lived, supervised by qualified local preceptors and visited periodically by faculty. Education and administration courses could be taken at other universities. Classes were scheduled at alternating hours (evenings one semester, mornings the next), and, if possible, several courses were taught in one day, decreasing the number of days the students would have to be away from their jobs. Courses were also taught off campus, and occasionally an interactive video format was used to teach nursing courses originating on campus to students living in St. Petersburg and Fort Myers.

The master's program at Oklahoma was planned for working students. Classes were offered on the main campus and at an extension program established in Tulsa. Students came from Oklahoma, Kansas, and Arkansas, and one coming from a distance traveled weekly by plane to attend. Students completed all their work in one day each week, the days lasting from ten in the morning until six in the evening. They could earn as many as eight credits a semester by attending the one day each week.

The rural and mountainous nature of many of the eight surrounding states served by the Knoxville project made it unique in the scope of its outreach. Four satellite class locations—Chattanooga, Kingsport, and Cookeville, Tennessee; and Lexington, Kentucky—were arranged to meet the needs of students from the large geographical area, but still over half of the students had to commute more than sixty miles to their classes. For some, a drive of five hours or more to reach class was necessary. Some of these nurses lived in reasonable proximity to a city where there was an existing MSN program, but classes in these programs were not scheduled to accommodate working students. This alarming fact may be of future consequence in the preparation of teachers for ADN programs.

The off-campus courses had several distinctive qualities. First, the course objectives were introduced in an intensive workshop-seminar at the beginning of the quarter, on a Friday or a Saturday. The instructor provided an overview of the basic concepts, distributed bibliographies and learning modules or packets, and gave assignments to be completed before the next meeting of the class.

Next, a second seminar was held at midquarter. During this class meeting, midterm papers and projects were submitted, and a variety of experiential and didactic learning activities took place.

Finally, a third session at the end of the quarter included final examinations or the submission of culminating course projects or term papers.

Between class meetings, students viewed videotapes at the satellite locations and used other learning materials developed specifically for them. Learning modules were available for twelve courses: nine graduate courses and three courses designed for individuals who had nonnursing baccalaureate degrees or who had not taken the prerequisites for specific graduate courses.

These modules were used in various ways: to supplement textbooks and classroom lectures, to assist the student in self-paced independent study, and to provide a way (through assignments to be mailed back to the instructor) for faculty to evaluate student progress. Instructors were available by collect telephone calls for consultation, and project newsletters disseminated updated information at regular intervals.

Students

The majority of the students attending project programs had considerable teaching and clinical experience at the time they enrolled; 65 percent were currently teaching, 54 percent in an ADN program. Two-thirds of them had three or more years of teaching experience. Because these teachers had not had access to graduate programs in nursing, 19 percent had matriculated with a master's or a doctoral degree in another discipline, usually education. Moreover, 67 percent had six or more years of clinical practice experience, usually in medical-surgical nursing (80 percent).

It may be somewhat surprising, therefore, to learn that the most important goals of these students were to improve their teaching ability (84 percent) and to update their clinical practice skills (83 percent). The additional reasons they gave for matriculating included enhancing their personal development (76 percent), increasing their opportunity for job advancement (75 percent), and increasing their job security (67 percent). More immediate goals included learning how better to develop curricula (68 percent), construct tests (55 percent), create learning materials (54 percent), and assess the clinical performance of their students (50 percent).

In Oklahoma, as an example, eight teachers from one ADN program were enrolled; their continued employment depended on their making substantial progress toward the MSN. Of all the students in the program, 87 percent were working. Like others in the project, they typically were single parents, some were experiencing illness in the family, and most were struggling with heavy teaching loads.

Students at all the sites across the country identified stress and self-pressure as being a matter of great concern to them. They, very like the students they were teaching in basic nursing programs, were concerned about juggling role responsibilities—worker, student, family provider, and caretaker—and managing their time wisely. Their faculty noted that some were carrying heavy loads but viewed them as mature and highly motivated.

In California, students' anxiety peaked at two points: the first wave occurred upon their entering the program and the second upon their beginning their field experience. The support offered by faculty members, mentors, and preceptors at these times lessened the stress.

The students handled the extraordinary pressures deftly. They formed study groups and telephone networks to supplement class work, as classes were held less frequently in this program than in traditional programs. They took advantage of their status as long-distance commuters by carpooling and using travel time for discussions of goals and concerns. They shared resources and solutions generously with one another.

In addition, newsletters issued regularly linked the students participating in the project in different locations; and an "MSN Telephone Bulletin Board," a recorded message service, instituted in California in 1986, provided callers with updated information on upcoming classes and other events.

Despite the fact that all the students' employers had declared themselves in support of their participation, few actually made concessions in their teaching assignments, except for making minor schedule changes. In the face of the resulting pressures on their time and energy, the students showed a strong commitment to advancing their own education, persevering in the master's program and, often, declaring their intention to proceed with doctoral study.

The students' employers often did behave paradoxically, urging them on the one hand to complete the requirements for the master's degree but making few concessions regarding released time for attending classes or fulfilling clinical and teaching practice hours. The students had to arrange for their own replacements when their own teaching schedules conflicted with scheduled clinical days in the master's program. One student enrolled in the Tennessee program was forced to terminate her program because her director, after promising her the summer off so that she could complete her clinical practice, reneged at the last moment, just weeks before the start of the summer quarter. Less disastrous but more common was students' having to take courses out of sequence because of the inflexibility of their own teaching schedules.

Virtually all of the students in the California program worked full-time and had family responsibilities. The majority were married (94 percent), had children (75 percent), and were younger than forty (69 percent). Most lived in southern California fairly near the sites for classes, but a few students commuted long distances from northern California to attend seminars. (Airfare, motels, and other travel expenses made the program quite costly for these nurses.) The willingness of the students to assume the costs, both literal and figurative, of participating in the program attests to the desirability of a nontraditional program for preparing ADN teachers.

The student group in Nebraska were somewhat younger than those at other project sites (90 percent were under age forty), and they were more likely to be rearing children (89 percent had children under twelve years old) and to be less experienced in ADN education (only 32 percent claimed ADN teaching experience). The majority were part-time students (61 percent) and commuted thirty miles or less to their graduate classes (72 percent).

Students who enrolled in the Florida program were primarily married women with children who worked full-time or part-time while pursuing graduate study. Florida students were older than students elsewhere in the project; half were over the age of forty, and four of them were older than fifty. One of the students in the over-fifty category, already a junior college faculty member, received the prestigious Outstanding Student in USF Award—determined by faculty vote—at the December 1986 commencement.

Although there were six students from Iowa at the Nebraska site, the majority of the fifty-two students enrolled were Nebraska residents. A higher percentage of Iowa students had been expected, but many community colleges in Iowa as well as Nebraska were experiencing financial difficulty because of the farm crisis of the time, and faculty members could obtain released time for graduate study only with great difficulty.

In Tennessee the majority of the students were female (98 percent), under age forty (77 percent), and married (74 percent). Most had children (77 percent). Virtually all had teaching experience, 65 percent having taught in ADN programs and 26 percent in diploma programs. Several students were ADN or diploma program directors. Students were more likely to reside in rural (46 percent) or suburban (24 percent) communities than in urban areas (30 percent). Many were faculty members in junior colleges located in relatively isolated regions such as the hills of West Virginia, rural Alabama and Georgia, the economically depressed areas of Tennessee and Kentucky that once were booming coal-mining locales, and in small North Carolina communities across the mountains from Knoxville.

The willingness of faculty everywhere in the program to accommodate program entrants who did not hold the BSN exhibits a flexibility that is often lacking in graduate nursing education, with unfortunate results. A cadre of highly capable and motivated individuals over the years have acquired bachelor's degrees in other disciplines when no BSN or MSN programs were accessible to them, technically meeting the requirements that enable them to teach in ADN programs but earning credentials that otherwise have very little value to them. The consequent loss to the nursing discipline is incalculable.

Among the applicants to programs at all the sites there was considerable diversity of academic ability. Several potential students did not meet the admission criteria of an undergraduate B average and an average aptitude on the Graduate Record Examination (GRE). They were admitted provisionally and offered assistance in their effort to achieve degree-seeking status. In Florida, for example, if such students' performance in the initial core courses proved to be satisfactory, they were admitted to the program; most of them were able to fulfill all requirements and earn their degrees. A few of these students showed exceptional intellectual ability. Several of these persons in Florida received highly competitive University Graduate Council Fellowships, which are awarded on the basis of high scores on tests of academic aptitude.

Transitional programs for students who were enrolled in the master's program but who did not hold the baccalaureate degree were offered, and these were greatly welcomed by the students. In fact, they were considered essential for the success of the overall project. In California, for example, students could have their undergraduate transcripts evaluated and then take undergraduate courses to fill any gaps that were discovered. In Florida, students were allowed to take physiology, statistics, physical assessment, and research courses or to challenge these courses by examination to acquire baccalaureate equivalency. Several prepared for the challenge examinations by independent study.

Each project site had stipends to be awarded to students recommended for assistance by the faculty. Of all the students enrolled nationally, 51 percent were concerned about their ability to pay for their participation in the program. Although this level of concern is lower than the level of concern regarding stress and conflicting demands, it is high enough to make it clear that the availability of financial assistance was reassuring to students.

The faculties at the six sites distributed stipends differently, but generally the money was used to pay tuition and fees. In Florida, for example, the money for tuition and fees was given to forty-six part- and full-time students, and students having greater needs were awarded more. Small grants were also made to students traveling 300 miles or more, to cover the cost of travel. In Oklahoma, tuition and fees were paid in the first year, and during the second year monies were added for travel costs for students coming from long distances. At the Nebraska site, stipends were used to pay tuition for nine credit hours each semester, for a maximum of thirty-nine credit hours of study for each student.

Stipends were particularly appealing to students who were young single parents juggling many role responsibilities. In Florida, faculty reported that students considered the money a measure of their worth; it became a strong element in their motivation to complete the project and succeed in their careers. Faculty members believed that the money, in most cases $400 to $500 a semester, did not solve financial needs so much as it provided an important psychological boost for a good performance.

In Oregon and Tennessee the selection of students who would receive stipends was made by advisory groups. The student, after being admitted to degree candidacy, could apply for financial assistance. Preference was given to applicants who were currently teaching in ADN programs, who had average scores on a standard graduate test, who had undergraduate grades of B or better, and, in Tennessee, who were teaching in programs not yet accredited by the NLN. Usually these programs were located in rural areas that were having difficulty recruiting qualified faculty.

Stipends were disbursed directly to the students in increments, contingent upon satisfactory progress through the program. Some students who received project funds also received federal traineeship money, financial support from employers, and scholarships. Forty-five students were awarded stipends in Tennessee, and a comparable number received assistance at the other sites.

A Unique Program for ADN Faculty: The Issues

The broadest question addressed by the project was whether a special master's program to prepare ADN faculty is necessary. Proponents of

ADN education argued affirmatively, using as a model the educational preparation for elementary and secondary school teaching. The faculty in the graduate nursing program argued just as vehemently that a special program is not needed, as the standard program could easily be adapted to serve the needs of all students preparing to teach at any level in the system.

The graduate faculty contended that the principles and the processes are the same, regardless of the eventual educational goal. They argued that subspecialization is especially handicapping to the student. A special course on technical nursing or the adaptation of an existing course would suffice to meet the need, they said. Further, a desire for clinical certification in a specialty area strained the student and the program beyond the breaking point. Evaluations of the program by students gave the nod to the graduate educators: in their opinion, a program at the master's level especially for the preparation of ADN faculty is not a necessary prerequisite for teaching in the ADN program. An adaptation of a program already in existence as the best answer was shown by the project's experience.

What is of particular interest is how the master's program was modified to accommodate the learner preparing to teach in the ADN program.

In Tennessee a needs assessment survey to identify applicants' specific educational goals was undertaken. The survey instrument was distributed to fifty-five nursing schools in eight states — Tennessee, Kentucky, Georgia, Alabama, North Carolina, South Carolina, Virginia, and West Virginia.

The survey asked for interest in topics covered in the existing master's curriculum and for choices of clinical concentrations. The curriculum for a new track for ADN educators was developed partially on the basis of the responses. It included the two clinical concentrations desired by the proponents of ADN education since the 1960s. It also included an entirely new course specifically addressing the history of and contemporary issues in technical nursing and nursing education, and the proper use of teaching strategies for the adult learner in the community college.

The new track consisted of sixty quarter hours, including the following components: twenty-three hours of core courses, including courses on current health issues, nursing theories, behavioral dynamics, statistics, pathophysiology, nursing research, and a seminar on leadership strategies; twelve hours of clinical courses; nineteen hours of education courses; and six hours of electives. A master's thesis was not required, but those students wishing to complete a thesis as a part of their program substituted the thesis for the elective course hours. An unusually high number (more than half) of students in the project chose the thesis option.

Five new courses were developed specifically for the ADN educator track. The first was a four-hour theory course that examined human responses to deviations from wellness and explored effective nursing interventions for selected health problems. The next three were practice offerings that focused on the students' clinical interests. Adult nursing, maternal-child health, and psychosocial nursing courses were put together especially for the ADN teacher. And finally, a five-hour course highlighting the philosophy, history, and contemporary issues in technical nursing and nursing education was developed.

Students commuted to, or lived in, Knoxville for a summer session devoted to the clinical segment of the program. The clinical courses were designed to expose the students to the state-of-the-art theory and practice in selected clinical specialty areas, and they included sixteen hours of clinical practice each week. Students' evaluations of the clinical courses were very positive, attesting to the value of their experiences in the diverse institutions of a metropolitan medical center. This was especially valuable experience for the students from small rural communities.

The educational component of the track to prepare ADN teachers included the following:

Educational theories, philosophies	3 hours
Curriculum planning, development	3 hours
Education courses of student's choice (administration, computer applications, etc.)	3 hours
Teaching strategies, practicum	5 hours
Directed study in technical nursing education	5 hours
	19 hours

The first three of these courses could be taken at other universities. The remaining two were taught by the nursing faculty at satellite locations. Students did their practice teaching in an ADN program other than their employing institution, with supervised opportunities for providing both classroom and clinical instruction. They were exposed to the day-to-day operations of the nursing program, attended faculty meetings, and observed other instructors in the classroom and the clinical area.

The capstone course of the education concentration enabled the student to trace the history of the ADN program from its origin, to explain the current mission of the nursing program in the community college, to identify the unique characteristics of the adult learner and their consequences for teaching, and to describe the role of the technical nurse and the philosophical premises upon which this role is based. The analysis of selected critical issues that affect AD nursing programs and their graduates encouraged students to articulate their own philosophy of ADN education and practice. Students were then able to develop an AD nursing program of study consistent with the philosophy and conceptual framework they had just formulated.

The results of pre- and posttest studies of students' beliefs and attitudes regarding the differentiation of technical and professional categories of nursing, the articulation of ADN and BSN programs, the appropriate practice settings for ADN graduates, the credentials and preparation of ADN faculty, and other pertinent topics addressed in the course revealed considerable changes by the end of the course. Many students stated that they had never been exposed to Mildred Montag's initial formulation of technical nursing education before seeing the videotape on the subject in the course. Others admitted that they had tried to teach students all *they* knew, without gearing their instruction for the ADN students specifically.

The curricular revision of the master's program at other sites was less extensive but just as important. Generally, the curricula at all project sites were of similar design. They ranged in credit hours between sixty quarter hours and thirty-six to forty-one semester hours, but the purposes and direction of all were the same.

At Portland two new courses were created and an existing one was revised to meet the needs of ADN teacher students. The individuals responsible for developing, modifying, and teaching these courses described their initial impressions of the students as they began the coursework. As in Tennessee, many of them had no previous education courses, despite many years of experience teaching in community colleges. They had been designing courses but had no overall conceptual framework as the basis. They were also unaware of some of the critical differences between ADN and BSN education. For example, some of the students believed that "the ADN program prepares the same nurse as the BSN program; it is just done in two years." Students at other sites also held this belief.

At the outset of the course the ADN educator-students were anxious. Lacking the master's degree, they were afraid for their positions. In turn, this caused feelings of anger, frustration, and a certain amount of insecurity. Portland faculty goals for the course were to increase the students' knowledge about nursing and course development, moving them from doing what they did instinctively to thinking conceptually about course design.

A measurement and evaluation course met a need that was recognized early on by both the students and the educators. Most of the ADN teachers had learned on the job about the mechanics of creating, for example, multiple-choice tests and clinical evaluation tools. They were unacquainted with the theoretical basis for measurement and had received no formal instruction in the preparation of educational objectives, outcomes, and tests.

The instructor of the measurements course had taught the ADN teacher-students in an on-campus research course during the first summer of the program. The experience provided him with (1) knowledge of their previous coverage of statistics and other topics pertinent to the measurement and evaluation course, and (2) knowledge of the students as individual learners. Knowing the students personally was vital, considering the unique delivery system for this course. It was taught during the academic year, when students had left the Portland campus and returned to their homes throughout the United States. Nine learning modules, designed for self-paced study, were prepared for the students to work with at home. Contact with the faculty member and feedback regarding the required assignments was by telephone. The instructor spoke with each student on the average of once a week. The time spent in these telephone consultations and in grading papers was roughly comparable to the time that might have been spent in conventional class meetings. One advantage of this method over the traditional classroom method was the individualized nature of the instruction.

A further advantage was that, as they took the course, students could apply what they were learning directly in their own work, with their own students. This also worked to the advantage of the instructor of the third course in the sequence. This course, focused on teaching strategies for adult learners, was also taught during the academic year while students were not present on the Portland campus.

This course was unusual in that students participated through audio-teleconferencing ten times during the semester, during evening hours. These sessions usually began with a brief period for personal exchanges among students as they connected on-line through the AT&T bridge, followed by a twenty- to thirty-minute lecture by the instructor and a lively discussion among class members, all of whom knew one another from previous classes together. The instructor had noted that it was helpful for him to have taught the students in an adult growth and development course earlier in their program of study.

The focus of the course was on the psychology of the classroom and the nature of good teaching. One goal of the course was to move students beyond a narrow, vocational approach to teaching, to a consideration of the larger philosophical issues in education. Mortimer Adler's ideas were introduced at the beginning of the course, prompting students to search out the relevant writings in the great literature of the Western tradition. Students were also required to complete a major project that was pragmatic and job-related. Here, too, the opportunity for students to apply what was being learned directly to their work was an important element in the success of the course.

The course may need to be modified in the future, to cut the costs of audio-teleconferencing. Lectures may be taped instead and made available for rent or purchase by the students, so that on-line time can be devoted entirely to class discussion. Other innovations are being considered.

In Nebraska students pursuing the ADN education track enrolled in a three-hour curriculum course, a three-hour course on teaching in schools of nursing, and a practicum that gave students experience teaching in an ADN program. The curricular purposes were identical to those of other project sites.

The central feature of the curriculum course was a group project requiring students to act as a faculty to develop their own ADN curriculum. Each student then individually developed one of the courses described in the overall curricular plan. As in other projects, students discussed and explored the differences in ADN, BSN, and hospital-based nursing education programs.

In the teaching course, students were provided two video cameras and a monitor to record classes as they taught them and postconferences as they conducted them. The taping made it possible for them and for others to evaluate their performance as teachers. In addition, five learning modules were developed for use in the course. These addressed the legal aspects of the teaching role, test construction, and various aspects of career development for nurse educators, including job search and interviewing skills.

The curriculum at Oklahoma included core courses of ten credit hours directed toward nursing theory, a clinical practicum, and two cross-clinical seminars that may be elected in several clinical specialties. Supporting courses of ten to twelve credit hours included two research courses, a course in micro-teaching, a personal mastery seminar, and a course on the issues and management of health care systems. A leadership course was required, along with four credit hours of a functional pathway in education, management, or clinical specialization. Six to nine credit hours were taken outside the college of nursing. At the end, a comprehensive examination or a thesis was written.

Students enrolled in the project took a one-credit-hour course entitled "Special Studies in Associate Degree Education." Students could choose clinical studies in community health, maternity nursing, pediatric nursing, adult care nursing, and psychosocial nursing. They also engaged in projects to prepare course outlines, syllabi, test leveling, computer-assisted instructional (CAI) modules, audio and video tapes, and other instructional aids.

In California the curricular option that emphasized the role of the nurse educator included four units: foundations in nursing education, curriculum development, instructional design and evaluation, and strategies for teaching client care. Because there were many more ADN than BSN programs in California, the majority of the students selecting the nurse educator role were ADN faculty or were preparing for ADN positions. In the curriculum course the differences between ADN and BSN education were highlighted. One major assignment to students was to take a curricular framework and develop it from the ADN perspective.

In their performance courses the future ADN educators learned to prepare learning materials and to implement a teaching plan for a group of ADN students, both under the supervision of a preceptor. They also provided clinical instruction, which was evaluated by the preceptor. The final course in this performance segment required students to analyze the forces shaping nursing education, to explore the various aspects of faculty responsibilities (e.g., serving on standing committees of the university), and to formulate their own plans for self-evaluation and personal growth.

In a simulation seminar, the students who had chosen to focus on the educator or the administrator role worked together in fictitious joint appointments to deal with issues of mutual concern—health care trends, work-role definitions, ethical dilemmas, quality assurance programs. This segment of the program was particularly beneficial in providing the participants the opportunity to match an educator's with an employer's expectations, and to develop a better appreciation of each other's roles and viewpoints. The seminar gave the participants good experience on which to base future conduct in an area that has given nursing great difficulty—achieving a good fit between the AD nurse's education and her work role as defined by her initial employer (see chapter 10).

The question whether ADN teacher students should concentrate educationally in more than one clinical specialty area has been particularly acute for students in the Florida project. The goal of two clinical specialty concentrations is strongly supported by advocates of the ADN program but presents undue hardships for the students and the faculty in the graduate program. The state of Florida has specific certification requirements that differ from those of the ANA for each area of specialty practice but that must also be met before nurses can become certified in the state. Certification is important to nurse educators in order that they may maintain a private clinical practice and provide consultation services alongside their teaching responsibilities. Consequently, the graduate program in Tampa is built with a strong clinical specialty component.

Students preparing to be ADN teachers were also desirous of meeting the certification requirements through their program of study. Many of them were excited at getting back into clinical work, not only updating rusty skills but frequently pursuing entirely new areas of practice. In many cases, meeting the requirements necessitated the addition of coursework and clinical practice hours to the specified curriculum to prepare the ADN teacher. Some were willing to go beyond the specified number of hours in a given clinical concentration in order to enrich their theory base and improve their clinical abilities in the chosen area. The question that can be asked is whether the clinical certification in a specialty area is necessary for the student preparing to teach in the ADN program.

Concluding Thoughts

The most evident result of the project was the increased understanding of the differences between ADN and BSN education on the part of all who participated. They achieved a more complete grasp of the philosophical issues and the historical background that explains how the issues arose. Interestingly, many of the ADN educators who were students in the project changed positions, coming to the conviction that the BSN should be required for entry into professional practice and that the expectations of ADN students should be scaled down to the level described in the original Cooperative Research Project. The students' political awareness regarding the complex issues of licensure and titling, as well as other issues in nursing, was greatly heightened by the program.

Consensus about the roles of associate degree and baccalaureate nurses in hospitals evolved from meetings of advisory groups working the master's programs. As a result of the project activity, networking among people in ADN and MSN facilities was established, and the educational offerings in both improved. The controversy over the entry-into-practice policy positions of the national nursing organizations may well continue, but at the grass-roots level the project developed new understandings and working relationships.

Associate degree nurse educators, mostly directors of programs, were asked to participate on advisory committees, which in some cases also included nursing service directors and junior college administrators. These committees discussed issues, recommended placement sites for students, and sometimes determined which students were to receive financial assistance. Often they commented on course design and recommended specific content that would be most helpful to the ADN program they represented.

The faculty of the College of Nursing in Oklahoma and an advisory group to the project believed that teaching in ADN programs in the project area improved as a result of the project's work. The advisory group reported changed behavior among faculty who were in school, as well as curricular improvements and a general elevation of standards and expectations. The five associate degree program directors on the committee did not want to terminate the group at the project's end. Junior college groups from Arkansas and Kansas reported similar responses.

The cadre of program graduates who have returned to, or obtained, positions in ADN education already positively influence these schools. Several are serving as preceptors for other students who are doing teaching practicums. ADN directors have been supportive of the program and have encouraged their faculty members who do not hold the MSN to enroll. The reputation of the programs has also attracted several people who have taken the teaching track as post-master's students.

The Tampa site director considered the Kellogg project her most satisfying professional experience. Universally, faculty praised the students for their accomplishments. Some at first had questioned whether they should be involved with a project designed to assist the ADN movement. As the projects neared completion, all were convinced that the master's program had contributed to an improvement of teaching generally, and particularly in lessening the tensions between ADN and BSN educators. A Portland teacher felt that the project's graduates had become a positive influence on the ADN movement. "We have graduated a more broadly prepared educator," she declared, "and we've touched many lives." Project students presenting their work at various agencies and at meetings convey a positive model that reflects well on the project. Research interests have been awakened, and students are seeking ways to apply the results of their research to their work.

Finally, the projects provided an opportunity for a few students to obtain a master's education who otherwise could not have done so without financial assistance. Federal funds were scarce and other help was reserved for the gifted, which meant that this project filled a large gap in the array of available assistance.

Epilogue

The ADN program has made a substantial contribution to the shape of American nursing of the late 1980s. Born in the nursing shortage crisis of the late 1950s and early 1960s, the educational program graduated more than half of all RNs in the class of 1983.[1] That year 37 percent of all RNs working in hospitals were AD graduates, and the percentage was growing.[2] The ADN program has been firmly established within the educational system and is loyally supported across the country by the junior colleges that are its home.

The ADN movement has been highly successful. Its teachers have demonstrated new teaching practices and have dared to differ with the conventional educational wisdom of the day. Its programs have moved novice education for nurses from the service-based hospital whose mission is patient care to the general system of education in this country. Nursing education is now paid for in tax dollars rather than patient-care dollars. This goal, along with the establishment of a more educational environment for students learning to become nurses, was formulated in the early postwar years, was embraced by all concerned, and is now nearly accomplished, thanks in no small part to associate degree education.

The program has recruited students for nursing who would otherwise have chosen different careers. Men, married women with children, minority students, and others elected the AD program when other programs had more restrictive admission criteria or required long hours of clinical practice instruction. ADN faculty distinguished themselves in educating the disadvantaged learner. ADN education has provided the opportunity for career mobility to students who wish to further their education; a few ADN graduates now hold doctorates in disciplines related to nursing.

ADN education has brought the strengths of the American junior and community college educational system to a practice discipline long associated with apprentice training. Nurse educators adjusted well to the junior college milieu, and junior college faculty and administrators have adjusted some of their long-held beliefs and practices to accommodate the nursing curriculum. The marriage has been a long and happy one.

The ADN program has enjoyed strong foundation support through the years, in part because of the initiative of faculty who sought funds and in part because of the foundations' effort to seek solutions for the chronic nursing shortage. Federal monies were also available to ADN programs willing to admit more nursing students, to keep open programs in the face of financial distress, or to begin new programs to alleviate local nursing shortages.

If one achievement could be singled out as being the most crucial contribution ADN education has made to health care delivery in this country today and in the foreseeable future, it would have to be its role in alleviating the nursing shortage since the program's inception in the middle 1950s. Today yet another crisis in the supply of nurses is of concern to health policymakers. It is estimated that approximately 11.3 percent of all nursing positions are vacant. In May 1988 the American Hospital Association reported that three of four hospitals were relying on overtime of their current staff to fulfill their service needs. Nearly half of the hospitals employed temporary or agency nurses to combat shortages, and many hospitals, most of them on the East Coast, have employed foreign nurses. Beds have been closed and emergency departments shut down.[3]

Enrollments in nursing programs began a steep decline in 1983 and have not returned to their base levels. By 1986 an overall decline of 7.8 percent was noted, and the situation is worsening each year. In 1987 the AACN reported a 9.2 percent drop in enrollments in baccalaureate programs, and enrollment figures from hospital-based schools and ADN programs have shown an even greater decline.[4] According to a report released by U.S. Department of Health and Human Services in 1986, the number of newly licensed RNs will drop 15.6 percent by the year 2000.[5]

Nursing schools overall are graduating fewer nurses. In 1986 82,000 nurses graduated, but by 1987 the number was down to 77,000. Fewer applicants are matriculating to nursing schools. There were 46,000 in 1984 and only 34,000 two years later.[6]

Contributing to the problem of declining enrollments is the size of the college-age population, which has been dropping steadily since 1981. The current college population will decline from 30.5 million to about 27 million before it bottoms out in 1995, at which time it is expected to start growing again.[7]

Among freshman women, the population of potential nurses has dropped 51 percent since 1974, according to Kenneth C. Green, associate director of the Cooperative Institutional Research Program at UCLA, who culled the information from the program's annual survey of 275,000 college freshmen. The ratio of future nurses to prospective women physicians dropped from just over 3 to 1 in 1968 to just under 1 to 1 in 1986. In light of the fact that about 95 percent of nursing students are women, Green estimated that by 1990 the nation's colleges are likely to award more medical degrees than baccalaureate nursing degrees to women.[8] Dean Gail Harkness of Boston University School of Nursing has said that by the year 2000, 40 percent of the nation's pharmacists, 21 percent of its physicians, and 16 percent of its dentists are expected to be women.[9]

The number of male and minority students choosing nursing is quite low. In 1978 only 6.3 percent of nursing students were men or minorities. Eight years later the number had increased slightly, to 6.6 percent. But the number of men in nursing is still "the all-time most dramatic" example of gender underrepresentation of any occupational group, worse than the lack of female participation in law enforcement, fire fighting, and other traditionally male careers.[10]

The demand for nurses has never been greater. Hospitalized patients are sicker than ever before and demand care that is often associated with complex technology requiring higher nurse-patient ratios. The frail elderly population is becoming more numerous and demands increasing nursing time in hospitals. Cutbacks in auxiliary personnel have increased the need for more nurses, and competition for nursing personnel from agencies other than hospitals is a leading problem.

Nurses in hospitals are seeking jobs in surgicenters, HMOs, insurance companies, ambulatory care centers, corporations that use nursing expertise, and home health care agencies. In fact, home health care agencies are now beginning to attract critical care or other highly skilled specialty nurses because they offer working conditions that are less stressful than hospital intensive care units.

An increasingly ill hospital population has produced several paradoxes related to the current shortage. James Gallaher, senior research associate at ANA, has pointed to several.

– The number of RNs is increasing at the same time that the number of patient days in hospitals is decreasing. In 1984 there were 375 million in-patient days compared with 332 million just three years later. The number of full-time equivalent nurses increased from 771,000 to 817,000 during the same period. The shorter hospital stay caused the patient acuity level to rise and thereby created a need for more nurses.
– The RN-to-patient ratio is increasing, again because of the patient acuity level. In 1977 there were 64 nurses for every 100 patients. Today there are 97 for every 100 patients. Patients require more intensive care usually associated with complex technology and stay shorter periods of time in the hospital.
– Contrary to popular belief, the number of nurses working in hospitals is increasing. "More than 75 percent of staff nurses are employed working in hospitals, more than ever before." But these nurses are subject to drop-out because of job-related stress, low salaries, and the high physical demands of their positions.[11]

The nursing shortages in this country have been chronic since the end of World War II. There are periods of crisis, leading some observers to define the shortage as cyclical, but there have been few periods when all experts would agree that supply and demand were in balance. The last crisis occurred in 1980; the previous one occurred in the late 1950s and the 1960s. Nevertheless, most health care policy experts say that the current shortage is different and far more serious. They see no end in sight.

Three methods for solving the chronic nursing shortage have been used since the end of World War II, but each with limited success. The first has been to increase the number of students coming through the educational system. Traditionally this has been accomplished by student loans, scholarships, and financial aid to institutions having or wanting to start up new programs to educate nurses. In the case of the ADN program, the growth in the number of students and programs resulting from this approach has been remarkable.

The second means of remedying the nursing shortage has been to attract inactive nurses back to the work force. The most commonly used strategy is to offer short-term educational programs to refresh the nurses' skills and abilities. Another means of attracting inactive RNs back to work is to offer competitive salaries. At times, economic difficulty, whether individual or social, has accomplished the same purpose. In nursing the work force participation rate has grown from about 55 percent in 1960 to 76 percent in 1980, and it has risen even higher, to 80 percent, in recent years.[12] The ADN program has made a significant contribution to growth in the number of working nurses by admitting students who were older, married, and in many instances single parents. For many of these people, the ADN program was the first and only program to offer such opportunity.

The third remedy most often attempted is the creation of a nurse assistant to relieve the RN of tasks that can be safely performed by others with less education. This solution has been used repeatedly since the end of World War II, but with only partial success. The categories of nurse assistants thus created include LPNs, nurse's aides, ward clerks, ward managers, and others, some of whom have come and gone with the times. Most recently, the AMA has suggested yet a new category of assistant called "registered care technologists." The irony of this newest "solution" from the point of view of ADN educators and policymakers is that ADN education itself was designed to vastly reduce the need for nursing assistants.

A fourth solution being discussed with increasing frequency is unionization.[13] Current estimates indicate that some 6 million nonunion health care workers employed in American institutions and hospitals may expect over the next few years a substantial increase in union activity. It is doubtful that RNs will join any mass union movement, but isolated strikes supported by individual nurses are likely to reoccur. The unionization of nurses has been a concern not only of health care agencies but also of foundations and other supporters of nurses and their educational institutions.

None of these solutions has been shown to cure the chronic state of nurse shortage in the country. Obviously, the right solution is yet to be discovered. Apparently, more basic issues must be addressed if a solution is to be worked out.

On 27 May 1988 the DHHS secretary's Commission on Nursing presented an interim report to Secretary Otis Bowen of Health and Human Services. The commission had been asked to identify the factors contributing to the nursing shortage and to propose solutions. It attributed the nation's failure to supply nurses to meet the demand to several factors, most notably the increasing level of illness of hospitalized patients, increased federal staffing requirements, cutbacks in auxiliary personnel, shorter lengths of hospital stay, advances in technology, increases in the number of elderly patients, and new hospital cost-containment measures.

Other factors of equal importance included low wages for staff nurses, the lack of enough nurses with advanced educational preparation in nursing, the lack of RN retention programs in hospitals, inadequate management policies in several hospitals, and changing career opportunities for women.[14]

In June of 1988 the Federation of Nurses and Health Professions (FNHP) issued a report that was not essentially different. The report said, in part, that the data on the nursing shortage were startling. FNHP President Owley said that "because of the growing number of senior citizens, the continued spread of diseases like AIDS, advances in technology, and the decreasing number of women choosing to go into the health professions, the demand for health care services is outstripping the supply of trained, qualified workers. What this is leading to is a potentially devastating curtailment or even 'rationing' of services. Such actions will impact most heavily on the poor, the elderly, and individuals who rely on government services."[15]

The FNHP recommended several strategies that have been extensively explored in the chapters of this book. The FNHP wanted career ladders and career mobility programs, a job design that effectively uses existing personnel, stronger linkages between hospitals and the educational institutions preparing novices, and a complete evaluation of salary structures.[16]

The American Association of Colleges of Nursing (AACN) suggested in May of 1988 the following remedies: new staffing systems to increase the time the nurse spends with the patient, better use of auxiliary personnel, the retention of experienced nurses in hospitals, better use of informational systems, outreach educational programs, career mobility avenues, work-study programs, and financial assistance for students.[17]

The need for federal assistance to alleviate the shortage is again under consideration. On 19 May 1988 legislation to reauthorize nursing education programs under Title VIII of the Public Health Service Act was introduced. The bill, entitled the "Nursing Shortage Reduction and Education Extension Act of 1988," is the counterpart to Senator Edward Kennedy's Nursing Shortages Reduction Act of 1987. Although the bills are not identical, they provide for essentially the same level of funding.

When the Nurse Education Act was last reauthorized in 1985, the funding was aimed at graduate education. The proposed legislation continues that funding for nurse practitioners, nurse midwives, gerontological nurses, administrators, and researchers but also provides new authorization levels of undergraduate nursing scholarships. For the first time in five years, funds are being made available for a loan repayment program. The bill also addresses innovative hospital nursing practice models, long-term care nursing practice demonstrations, and nurse recruitment centers.[18]

Pamela Maraldo, NLN executive director, suggested in August 1987 that "Opportunities arise whenever there is a positive or negative sequence of events. Change in either direction creates a new receptivity in the market place. . . . The market for nurses in hospitals is in trouble, because other career opportunities are outpacing us in their overall appeal. But, ironically, this could be the greatest opportunity nursing has ever had."[19]

Beginning in the 1960s the ADN educational program made a large difference in the shortage crisis by graduating nurses in a shorter time than did other RN programs. Another such shot in the arm cannot be expected today, but ADN programs will continue to graduate as many nurses as their present structure permits.

What ADN faculty and graduates can do effectively is to pursue those remedies to the nursing shortage that have been described in this book or currently suggested by organized voluntary and governmental bodies addressing the crisis of nurse supply.

The FNHP's suggestion, for example, that the job design of nursing be restructured to effectively use existing personnel is likely to have a profound effect on the retention of RNs in hospitals. The work reported here has highlighted the necessity of employing nurses to work at the level of competence for which they have been educationally prepared. When they have worked together, faculty and service personnel have been able to reach agreement on the work role of the new graduate.

We have reported how hospital units have been established and operated on the basis of differentiated practice defined in terms of nurses' educational attainment. These units have proven highly desirable places of employment for both new and older graduates. What is clearly demonstrated is that burnout or demoralization is greatly lessened when employer expectations do not exceed the graduates' abilities.[20]

We have seen how clinical ladders and career mobility programs, also suggested by FNHP and AACN, have been successfully developed and put into operation. Closer links between hospitals and educational institutions preparing novices have also been established, with good results. Joint committees and appointments, preceptorships, and joint marketing activities have also been highly successful.

Financial incentives for nurses who improve their practice skills and abilities through advanced education should be instituted. In the early years of the ADN movement, graduates seldom sought additional formal education; they were content to upgrade their knowledge and abilities through on-the-job training and continuing education programs. Since 1979, however, the number of nurses holding the ADN degree who have later graduated from BSN programs has steadily increased, from 3,007 in 1979 to 4,585 in 1983, and the number is expected to grow substantially in the years ahead.[21]

It is noteworthy that the criterion-based model used to project nursing manpower needs that was developed by a panel of experts for the federal government has predicted that by the year 2000 there will be roughly one-half as many BSN and higher-degree nurses, one and one-third as many AD nurses, and one and one-half the LVNs and LPNs required to meet the conservatively estimated nursing personnel need. This represents a deficiency of 619,100 prepared at the baccalaureate and higher level; an excess of 296,900 prepared at the AD level, and an excess of 204,200 licensed vocational nurses.[22] It can be concluded from such data that the original view of the ADN program as a terminal one should be modified to include the original mission of the junior college to provide the first two years of a baccalaureate degree.

Furthermore, consideration must be given to career planning for ADN graduates who choose to work at different hospitals or other health agencies during their working life. Carefully designed benefit packages, salary differentials, and incremental increases for advances in education and increased clinical expertise, and flexible scheduling are absolutely essential if we are to relieve the nursing shortage.

The future role of the ADN graduate in health care is quite clear. The graduates of the two-year program will remain the most numerous employees of acute care hospitals. Some of the AD nurses may move to chronic or long-term health facilities, but their educational preparation best prepares them for general hospital practice. Consensus concerning the work role of the associate degree graduate has now been reached.

The early projects concerned with the ADN program were often focused on the preparation of teachers for two-year nursing students. Early concerns were directed to specialized programs of teacher preparation, attracting faculty to the effort, and providing continuing education for teachers already employed in the ADN effort. Financial assistance to those pursuing the graduate degree was therefore deemed essential. Federal traineeships and foundation funding were an important ingredient in this effort.

Current work indicates that concern in ADN education now rests with other issues. Student access to educational opportunities is paramount to success, and access involves the availability of both faculty and instructional materials. ADN educators have evinced a strong interest in the use of instructional technology—instructional modules, VCRs, CAI, audio-cassettes. And ADN education will continue to attract teachers partially because its pressures on faculty to publish or conduct research are lower than in baccalaureate and graduate nursing education. The emphasis in ADN programs is on teaching.

Financial assistance is a catalyst for attracting students to the MSN program, which supplies ADN faculty. Even small sums are effective in retaining the graduate student in the teacher preparation program. Federal assistance or endowments may prove equal to meeting the future need.

The effort of professional nursing organizations to label the AD graduate as a technician, an associate nurse, or an assistant to the professional nurse has subsided, though titles have not been decided upon yet. What remains of that drive is the efforts of state nursing organizations to legislate the 1965 ANA Position Paper. Deadlines have again been set, but successful achievement of the 1965 goals remains very much dependent upon what happens as a result of the crisis of nurse supply.

The future of AD nursing is bright. Its history is starred with accomplishments. The most notable is the movement of nursing education from privately controlled hospitals to the general education system of this country. Many health care policy experts believed that it could not be done. As our research has shown, this most fundamental of all changes in nursing education in the last half of the twentieth century was the result of the convergence of several trends. The associate degree in nursing seems to be an example of yet another idea in history whose time had come.

Notes

Chapter 1

1   Quoted by Mildred D. Montag, "The Associate Degree Nursing Program" (unpublished paper submitted to the author, 1986), p. 1.
2   The figures differ, depending on whose statistics are consulted and which variables apply. Among those counting the nurses were the various nursing associations, the National Nursing Council, the Women's Bureau in the Labor Department, the branches of the military, the USPHS and its sundry subdivisions, the Veterans Administration, and the AHA.
3   Philip A. Kalisch and Beatrice J. Kalisch, *The Advance of American Nursing*, 2nd ed. (Boston: Little, Brown, 1986), p. 504.
4   Ibid., p. 542.
5   Ibid., pp. 534–535.
6   Ibid., p. 537.
7   The column appeared, for example, in the *Washington Post*, 19 December 1944.
8   Kalisch and Kalisch, *American Nursing*, p. 583.
9   Ibid., p. 539.
10 Ibid.
11 Stella Goostray, *Memoirs: Half a Century in Nursing* (Boston Nursing Archives, Boston University Mugar Memorial Library, 1969), pp. 116–117, as cited in ibid., p. 502.
12 As quoted in ibid., p. 502. The organizations referred to by their acronyms are the ANA—American Nurses' Association, NOPHN —National Organization of Public Health Nursing, NLNE—National League for Nursing Education, NACGN —National Association of Colored Graduate Nurses, ACSN —Association of Collegiate Schools of Nursing, and ARCNS—American Red Cross Nursing Services.
13 Ibid., p. 504.
14 A. W. Goodrich, "Nursing and National Defense," *American Journal of Nursing* 42 (1942): 11–16.
15 A. C. Haupt, "Our War Nursing Program," *American Journal of Nursing* 42 (1942): 1381–1385.
16 Philip A. Kalisch and Beatrice J. Kalisch, *The Advance of American Nursing*, 1st ed. (Boston: Little, Brown, 1978), p. 471.
17 Kalisch and Kalisch, *American Nursing* (2nd ed.), p. 542.
18 For details, see Lucile Petry, "A Summing Up: The U.S. Cadet Nurse Corps," *American Journal of Nursing* 45 (1945): 1027–1028. See also her description of the curriculum in "How to Qualify Under the Act," *Modern Hospital* 61, no. 3 (1943): 60–61.

19 Kalisch and Kalisch, *American Nursing* (1st ed.), pp. 473–475.

20 Ibid., p. 488.

21 Lewis Thomas, "Medical Lessons from History," in *The Medusa and the Snail* (New York: Bantam Books, 1980), p. 136.

22 H. Thomas Ballantine, M.D., as quoted by Frank D. Campion, *The AMA and U.S. Health Policy Since 1940* (Chicago: Chicago Review Press, 1984), p. 21.

23 "Residency Training of Physician Veterans," *JAMA* 131 (1946): 1356, as quoted in ibid., p. 31.

24 See especially Jo Ann Ashley, *Hospitals, Paternalism, and the Role of the Nurse* (New York: Teacher's College Press, Columbia University, 1976).

25 For an analysis of the factors behind the shortage, see Peter I. Buerhaus, "Not Just Another Nursing Shortage," *Nursing Economics* 5 (November-December 1987): 267–279; and Kalisch and Kalisch, *American Nursing* (2nd ed.), chap. 15.

26 See Philip A. Kalisch and Beatrice J. Kalisch, *The Federal Influence and Impact on Nursing* (Hyattsville, Md.: U.S. Department of Health and Human Services, June 1980), p. 192. This report, written under contract to the Division of Nursing, is available from the National Technical Information Service (HRP-0900636).

27 ANA, *Facts About Nursing* (1946), pp. 8–9.

28 Kalisch and Kalisch, *American Nursing* (1st ed.), pp. 491–492, 497–498.

29 Donald E. Yett, *An Economic Analysis of the Nurse Shortage* (Lexington, Mass.: Lexington Books, 1975), p. 10.

30 ANA, *Facts About Nursing* (1951), p. 41.

31 U.S. Bureau of Labor Statistics, *The Economic Status of Registered Professional Nurses, 1946–47*, Bulletin No. 931 (Washington, D.C.: Government Printing Office, 1947).

32 See Ashley, *Hospitals, Paternalism, and the Role of the Nurse*, for an impassioned summary of the reasons RNs have criticized hospitals as educators and employers. Kalisch and Kalisch also discuss the problem: *American Nursing* (1st ed.), pp. 493–496 and passim; and Buerhaus analyzes the effect of the problem on nurse recruitment.

Chapter 2

1 Shirley H. Fondiller, *The Entry Dilemma: The National League for Nursing and the Higher Education Movement, 1952–1972*, League Exchange No. 132, NLN Publication No. 41–1896 (New York: NLN, 1983), p. 119.

2 National League for Nursing Education, "Principles Relating to Organization, Control, and Administration of Nursing Education" (New York, 1947), as quoted in Fondiller, *The Entry Dilemma*, pp. 14–15.

3 Commission on Hospital Care, *Hospital Care in the United States: A Study of the Function of the General Hospital, Its Role in the Care of All Types of Illness, and the Conduct of Activities Related to Patient Service, with Recommendations for Its Extension and Integration for More Adequate Care of the American Public* (New York: Commonwealth Fund, 1947).

4 Also represented on the council were the National Association of Practical Nurse Education, the Red Cross, the Army Nurse Corps, the Navy Nurse Corps, USPHS and a number of its subdivisions including the Children's Bureau, as well as other federal agencies such as the Veterans Administration Nursing Service and the Bureau of Indian Affairs. See Emory W. Morris, "General Director's Report," in W. K. Kellogg Foundation, "Bimonthly Reports of the Officers to the Board of Trustees" (Battle Creek, Mich.: foundation archives, February-March 1949), p. 1.

5 Ibid., p. 1.

6 Ibid., p. 2.
7 E. L. Brown, *Nursing for the Future: A Report Prepared for the National Nursing Council* (New York: Russell Sage Foundation, 1948).
8 Ibid., pp. 165–166 and passim.
9 Morris, "General Director's Report," pp. 3–4.
10 Ibid., p. 4.
11 Ibid.
12 Ibid., p. 5.
13 W. K. Kellogg Foundation, "Annual Report of the Officers of the W. K. Kellogg Foundation to the Members of the Foundation" (Battle Creek, Mich.: foundation archives, 1949–1950), pp. 125, 136.
14 Kellogg, "Annual Report," 1948–1949, p. 151; Kellogg, "Annual Report," 1949–1950, p. 140, recounts further details about the funding and organization of the committee.
15 "Annual Report," 1949–1950, p. 142.
16 "Annual Report," 1950–1951, p. 165.
17 Ibid., p. 166.
18 Fondiller, *Entry Dilemma*, p. 26.
19 Mildred Montag, "The Associate Degree Nursing Program" (unpublished paper submitted to the author, 1986); Kalisch and Kalisch (1st ed.), pp. 510–511.
20 L. Petry, M. Arnstein, and R. Gillan, "Surveys Measure Nursing Resources," *American Journal of Nursing* 49 (1949): 770–772.
21 M. West and C. Hawkins, *Nursing Schools at the Mid-Century* (New York: National Committee for the Improvement of Nursing Services, 1950).
22 Montag, "Associate Degree Program."
23 ANA, *Facts About Nursing*, 1957, p. 67.
24 Montag, "Associate Degree Program."
25 "Annual Report," 1949–1950, pp. 140–141.
26 Eli Ginzberg, *A Program for the Nursing Profession* (New York: Macmillan, 1948), p. vii.
27 "Annual Report," 1947–1948, p. 114.
28 For summary reports of the project, see ibid., pp. 110–124; "Annual Report," 1948–1949, pp. 134–135.
29 Fondiller, *Entry Dilemma*, pp. 69–72.
30 Ibid.
31 Ibid.
32 Montag, "Associate Degree Program."

Chapter 3

1 Mildred L. Montag, "The Associate Degree Nursing Program" (unpublished paper submitted to the author, 1986), p. [6], quoting from her own *Community College Education for Nursing*.
2 Montag, personal communication, at the meeting of the advisory committee of the present project on 3–5 October 1984, Chattanooga, Tenn.
3 Montag, "Associate Degree Nursing Program," p. [7].
4 Ibid., pp. [7–8].
5 The account that follows relies on several sources: Ralph R. Fields, *The Community College Movement* (New York: McGraw-Hill, 1962), pp. 19ff.; Newton Edwards and Herman G. Richey, *The School in the American Social Order*, 2nd ed. (Boston: Houghton Mifflin, 1963), pp. 642 and passim. On California especially see Frank B. Lindsay, "California Junior Colleges: Past and Present," *California Journal of Second-*

ary Education 22 (March 1947): 137–142; W. C. Eells, "Historical Development: California," *The Junior College* (Boston: Houghton Mifflin, 1931), chapter 4.

6   Fields, *Community College Movement,* pp. 27–28.

7   Ibid., and *Junior College Journal* 1938: 317.

8   Jesse Parker Bogue, *The Community College* (New York: McGraw-Hill, 1950), p. 356.

9   Fields, *The Community College Movement,* pp. 18–19.

10 Charles R. Monroe, *Profile of the Community College: A Handbook* (San Francisco: Jossey-Bass, 1972), p. 11.

11 Fields, *The Community College Movement,* pp. 24–27. See also Elbert K. Fretwell, Jr., *Founding Public Junior Colleges* (New York: Teachers College, Columbia University, 1954).

12 Fields, *The Community College Movement,* chapter 2.

13 Thomas Diener, *Growth of an American Invention: A Documentary History of the Junior and Community College Movement* (New York: Greenwood, 1986), p. 131.

14 President's Commission on Higher Education, *Establishing the Goals* (Washington, D.C.: Government Printing Office, 1947), 1:67.

15 Ibid., 1:69.

16 Ibid., 1:68.

17 Volume 2 of the commission's report, entitled *Equalizing and Expanding Individual Opportunity,* explores these ideas in some detail.

18 Commission, *Goals,* 1:68.

19 Diener, pp. 131–148. Ewing was the author of a key government report two years earlier: see O. R. Ewing, *The Nation's Health: A Report to the President* (Washington, D.C.: Government Printing Office, 1948). In assessing the state of health care in the United States, it proposed the expansion of the nursing force and nurse training, to produce 50 percent more nurses each year.

20 Montag, "Associate Degree Nursing Program," pp. [10–11].

21 Ibid., p. [15].

22 Data for the year 1954, in ANA, *Facts About Nursing* (1957).

23 Montag, "Associate Degree Nursing Program," p. [20].

24 Ibid., p. [22].

25 Ibid., p. [21].

26 Ibid.

27 Ibid., p. [22].

28 Alice R. Rines, "Associate Degree Nursing Education: History, Development, and Rationale," *Nursing Outlook* 25 (1977): 496–501.

Chapter 4

1   Virginia O. Allen, "Pioneering Curricular Innovations Contributed by Associate Degree Nursing Educators" (unpublished paper submitted to the author, 1986). This chapter is based on Allen's paper and is the source being used unless another is cited.

2   Ralph W. Tyler, *Basic Principles of Curriculum and Instruction* (Chicago: University of Chicago Press, 1949).

3   Benjamin S. Bloom, *Taxonomy of Education Objectives: Handbook I, Cognitive Domain* (New York: David McKay, 1956).

4   Robert F. Mager, *Preparing Educational Objectives* (Belmont, Calif.: Fearon Publishers, 1962).

5   Mildred L. Montag, *Education for Nursing Technicians,* as quoted by Allen, "Curricular Innovations," p. 4.

6 Faye G. Abdellah, Irene L. Beland, Alameda Martin, Ruth V. Matheney, *Patient-Centered Approaches to Nursing* (New York: Macmillan, 1961).

7 Ibid., p. 75. See also R. V. Matheney, B. Nolan, G. J. Griffin, J. Griffin, and A. Ehrhart, *Fundamentals of Patient-Centered Nursing* (St. Louis: Mosby, 1964). Parts of this text were developed under the curriculum development phase of the New York sector of the four-state ADN education project funded by the W. K. Kellogg Foundation.

8 Ruth V. Matheney, "Pre- and Post-Conferences for Students," *American Journal of Nursing* 69 (1969): 286–289.

9 Many success stories about the use of multiple assignments in ADN programs have been written up. The ADN program at Manatee Community College in Florida is well known not only for using this method but for conducting workshops on its use to orient faculty members from programs throughout the country. See Janet T. Galeener, "Multiple Assignment," in NLN, *Leadership for Quality*, report of a conference held by the Department of Associate Degree Programs, St. Louis, March 1966, Publication No. 12–1240 (New York: NLN, 1966), pp. 34ff. See also J. T. Galeener, "Group or Multiple Student Assignment," *Journal of Nursing Education* 5 (April 1966): 29–31.

10 Marie M. Seedor, *Programmed Instruction for Nursing in the Community College* (New York: Teachers College, Columbia University, 1963), p. 2.

11 Samuel N. Postlethwait, *An Integrated Approach to Learning* (Edina, Minn.: Burgess, 1964).

12 Crystal M. Lange, "Auto-Tutorial and Mobile-Tutorial Laboratory Techniques in Nursing Education," in NLN, *Leadership for Quality*, pp. 21–25. Lange's paper is also available separately from ERIC (no. ED 014 960).

13 Gerald J. Griffin, Robert E. Kinsinger, Avis J. Pitman, *Clinical Nursing Instruction by Television* (New York: Teachers College, Columbia University, 1965).

14 June Simpson, "The Walk-Around Laboratory Practical Examination in Evaluating Clinical Nursing Skills," *Journal of Nursing Education* 6 (1967): 23–26.

15 E.g., John C. Flanagan, "The Critical Incident Technique," *Psychological Bulletin* 51 (1954): 327–358; Carrie B. Lenburg, *The Clinical Performance Examination* (New York: Appleton-Century-Crofts, 1979).

Chapter 5

1 ANA, *Facts About Nursing* (1952), p. 62; (1970–1971), p. 94.

2 Nursing Advisory Committee, W. K. Kellogg Foundation, Addendum G, minutes of the meeting 21–22 November 1957, in "Bimonthly Reports of the Officers to the Board of Trustees" (Battle Creek, Mich.: foundation archives, January-February 1958), p. 1.

3 Nursing Advisory Committee, W. K. Kellogg Foundation, Addendum A, minutes of the meeting 22, 23, 24 August 1957, in "Bimonthly Reports of the Officers to the Board of Trustees" (Battle Creek, Mich.: foundation archives, September-October 1957), p. 1.

4 Ibid., p. 2.

5 Ibid.

6 Addendum G, "Bimonthly Reports of the Officers to the Board of Trustees" (January-February 1958), p. 3.

7 Ibid., p. 4.

8 U.S. Bureau of the Census, *Statistical Abstract of the United States*, 105th ed. (Washington, D.C.: Government Printing Office, 1984), p. 152; ANA, *Facts About Nursing* (1961), p. 100.

9   Addendum G, "Bimonthly Reports of the Officers to the Board of Trustees" (January-February 1958), p. 3.
10 NLN, Department of Diploma and Associate Degree Programs, *Planning for Nursing Education in a Community College*, League Exchange No. 32, Publication No. 16–703 (New York: NLN, 1958).
11 Nursing Advisory Committee, Addendum D, minutes of the meeting 30 June–1 July 1958, in "Bimonthly Reports of the Officers to the Board of Trustees" (Battle Creek, Mich.: foundation archives, July-August 1958), p. 2.
12 Ibid., p. 3.
13 Ibid.
14 Ibid., pp. 17–18.
15 W. K. Kellogg Foundation, Minutes of the 349th Meeting of the Board of Trustees, "Bimonthly Reports of the Officers to the Board of Trustees" (Battle Creek, Mich.: foundation archives, 16 June 1959), p. 2. The meeting was devoted entirely to foundation programs in the hospital and nursing fields.
16 Bernice Anderson, *Nursing Education in Community Junior Colleges: A Four-State, 5-Year Experience in the Development of Associate Degree Programs* (Philadelphia: J. B. Lippincott, 1966), p. 107.
17 Ibid., p. 108.
18 Florida Community College Council, *The Community Junior College in Florida's Future: Report to the State Board of Education* (Tallahassee: Florida State Board of Education, 1957).
19 For more on the planning process in Florida, see G. H. DeChow, "The Development of an Associate Degree Nursing Program," *Journal of Nursing Education* 1 (September 1962): 9–10, 33–36; and J. L. Wattenbarger, "Florida's Community Junior Colleges and Nursing Education," *Florida Nurse* 10, no. 1 (1962): 35–36.
20 W. K. Kellogg Foundation, "Associate Degree Programs in Nursing," in Nursing section of "Annual Program Reports to the Board of Trustees" (Battle Creek, Mich.: foundation archives, 1958–1959), p. 15.
21 Ibid., p. 16.
22 "Decision of Nursing: Summary of Current Programs," in ibid., p. vi.
23 See "Associate Degree Programs in Nursing" and "Decision of Nursing: Summary of Current Programs," pp. 16–19, in ibid.
24 "Associate Degree Programs in Nursing," in ibid., p. 16.
25 ANA, *Facts About Nursing* (1960), p. 74 and passim.
26 Mildred L. Tuttle, Minutes of the meeting 4–5 June 1959, Nursing Advisory Committee, Addendum B, in "Bimonthly Reports of the Officers to the Board of Trustees" (Battle Creek, Mich.: foundation archives, July-August 1959), pp. 2–3.
27 W. K. Kellogg Foundation, "Associate Degree in Nursing," in Nursing section of "Annual Program Reports to the Board of Trustees" (Battle Creek, Mich.: foundation archives, 15 May 1960), pp. 2–9.
28 Ibid., p. 4.
29 Anderson, *Nursing Education in Community Junior Colleges*, pp. 41–42.
30 Ibid., pp. 79–81.
31 Ibid., pp. 111–112.
32 [New York] Nurse Resources Study Group, University of the State of New York, *Needs and Facilities in Professional Nursing Education* (Albany, N.Y.: author, 1959); see especially chap. 4.
33 For lists of publications originating in the four-state project, see Anderson, *Nursing Education in Community Junior Colleges*, the bibliography, and the companion vol-

ume to the present book, *Associate Degree Nursing Education: An Historical Annotated Bibliography, 1942–1983* (Durham, N.C.: NLN and Duke University Press, 1990).

34   Kellogg, "Associate Degree in Nursing" (15 May 1960), pp. 14–18, describes the New York projects.

35   ANA, *Facts About Nursing* (1958).

36   Kellogg, "Associate Degree in Nursing" (15 May 1960), pp. 18–19.

37   Kellogg, "Associate Degree in Nursing," in Nursing section of "Annual Program Reports to the Board of Trustees (Battle Creek, Mich.: foundation archives, 15 May 1961), p. 12.

38   Kellogg, "Associate Degree in Nursing," in Nursing section of "Annual Program Reports to the Board of Trustees" (Battle Creek, Mich.: foundation archives, 15 May 1963), p. 13.

39   Ibid., pp. 13–14.

Chapter 6

1   Philip A. Kalisch and Beatrice J. Kalisch, *The Federal Influence and Impact on Nursing* (Hyattsville, Md.: U.S. Department of Health and Human Services, June 1980), p. 340. This report, prepared under contract to the Division of Nursing, is available from the NTIS (no. HRP 0900636).

2   U.S. Bureau of the Census, *Historical Statistics of the United States: Colonial Times to 1970* (Washington, D.C.: Government Printing Office, 1975), pt. 1, pp. 73, 74. Equivalent 1985 dollar amounts have been computed using the annual average of the consumer price index as found in U.S. Bureau of the Census, *Statistical Abstract of the United States*, 107th ed. (Washington, D.C.: Government Printing Office, 1987), p. 454. Rounded off to the nearest dollar.

3   Kalisch and Kalisch, *Federal Influence*, p. 340.

4   Ibid., p. 321.

5   Ibid., p. 340.

6   Ibid., p. 396.

7   Ibid., p. 339.

8   Ibid., p. 340.

9   Frances P. Bolton, "Crisis in Health Care: Report to Congress on the Nursing Shortage," *Hospital* 28 (April 1954): 83–85.

10   Kalisch and Kalisch, *Federal Influence*, pp. 241–244.

11   Ibid., pp. 244–246, 247, 248–249.

12   Ibid., p. 249.

13   Ibid., p. 271.

14   Ibid., p. 272.

15   Ibid., pp. 286–287.

16   For a discussion of the ANA's lobbying efforts in Washington over the years, see Mary Anderson Hardy, "The American Nurses' Association Influence on Federal Funding for Nursing Education, 1941–1984," *Nursing Research* 36, no. 1 (January-February 1987): 31–35.

17   For example, see U.S. Congress, House of Representatives, *Hearings Before a Subcommittee of the Committee on Interstate & Foreign Commerce, House of Representatives—Health Amendments Act of 1956 (Nurse and Public Health Personnel Training—Commission on Nursing Services)*, Hearings, 84th Cong., 2nd sess. (on H. R. 11549), 13, 14, 15 June (Washington, D.C.: Government Printing Office, 1956), transcribes testimony regarding both Titles I and II.

18   Kalisch and Kalisch, *Federal Influence*, pp. 293, 313.

19 Ibid., pp. 331ff.

20 Ibid., pp. 332–335; Philip A. Kalisch and Beatrice J. Kalisch, *The Advance of American Nursing*, 1st ed. (Boston: Little, Brown, 1978), p. 605.

21 Kalisch and Kalisch, *Federal Influence*, p. 333.

22 Ibid., pp. 334–335.

23 Ibid., p. 335.

24 Ibid., p. 336.

25 Ibid., p. 335.

26 Ibid., p. 337.

27 Ibid., p. 346.

28 U.S. DHEW, Office of the Surgeon General, *Toward Quality in Nursing: Needs and Goals*, PHS Publication No. 992 (Washington, D.C.: Government Printing Office, 1963).

29 Ibid., p. 33.

30 Kalisch and Kalisch, *American Nursing* (1st ed.), pp. 658–659. The commission that was eventually formed, directed by Jerome P. Lysaught, would issue the much-discussed Lysaught study. See Shirley H. Fondiller, *The Entry Dilemma: The National League for Nursing and the Higher Education Movement, 1952–1972*, League Exchange No. 132, NLN Publication No. 41–1896 (New York: NLN, 1983), p. 51.

31 Fondiller, *Entry Dilemma*, pp. 50–51.

32 Kalisch and Kalisch, *Federal Influence*, p. 346.

33 Ibid., p. 345.

34 Ibid., pp. 349–350.

35 Ibid., p. 349.

36 Ibid., p. 350.

37 Ibid., p. 349.

38 Ibid., p. 351.

39 Ibid., p. 358. The legislative history of the act is reviewed on pp. 352–358.

40 Quoted in ibid., p. 351.

41 See United States, An Act to Amend the Public Health Service Act to Increase the Opportunities for Professional Nursing Personnel, and for Other Purposes (Public Law 88–581), *Statutes at Large* 78 (1964): 908–919, for the text of the law; see U.S. Congress, Senate, Committee on Labor and Public Welfare, *Nurse Training Act of 1964*, Senate Report No. 88–1378 (Washington, D.C.: Government Printing Office, 1964), for an overview of the bill.

42 The texts of their statements are published in U.S. Congress, House of Representatives, Committee on Interstate and Foreign Commerce, Subcommittee on Public Health and Safety, *Nurse Training Act of 1964*, Hearings, 88th Cong., 2nd sess., 8–10 April (Washington, D.C.: Government Printing Office, 1964).

43 Kalisch and Kalisch, *Federal Influence*, p. 359.

44 Ibid., p. 358.

45 Ibid., pp. 361–362.

46 Ibid., p. 361. The fact sheets published by the government included: U.S. DHEW, *The Nurse Training Act of 1964*, PHS Publication No. 1154 (Washington, D.C.: Government Printing Office, 1965), which provided an overview of the provisions of the act. Other pamphlets in this series were *Professional Nurse Traineeship Program* (1154–1); *Project Grants for Improvements in Nurse Training* (1154–2); *Payments to Diploma Schools of Nursing* (1154–3); *Nursing Student Loan Program: Information for Schools* (1154–4); and *Construction Grants Program for Schools of Nursing* (1154–5). Updates were published in 1969.

47   U.S. DHEW, Public Health Service, *Nursing Education Facilities, Programing Considerations and Architectural Guide: Report of the Joint Committee on Educational Facilities for Nursing of the National League for Nursing and the Public Health Service*, PHS Publication No. 1180-F-1B (Washington, D.C.: Government Printing Office, 1964). The guide provided an overview of nursing education, followed by a breakdown by program type giving the characteristics, needs, goals, programming and space requirements, budget, and other considerations affecting architectural considerations.

48   Kalisch and Kalisch, *Federal Influence*, pp. 370–371.

49   ANA, *Facts About Nursing* (1970–1971), p. 94.

50   Fondiller, *Entry Dilemma*, p. 79.

51   *Report of the National Advisory Commission on Health Manpower* (Washington, D.C.: Government Printing Office, 1967), 1: 24, as quoted in Fondiller, *Entry Dilemma*, p. 41.

52   Ibid.

53   Kalisch and Kalisch, *Federal Influence*, p. 422.

54   U.S. DHEW, *Nurse Training Act of 1964: Program Review Report*, PHS Publication No. 1740 (Washington, D.C.: Government Printing Office, December 1967).

55   Kalisch and Kalisch, *Federal Influence*, pp. 403–404, summarizes the recommendations.

56   Ibid., p. 398.

57   Ibid., p. 399.

58   Ibid., p. 418. For the text of the act, see United States, An Act to Amend the Public Health Service Act to Extend and Improve the Programs Related to the Training of Nurses . . . (Public Law 90–490), *Statutes at Large* 82 (1968): 773–789. For testimony of nursing leaders during the various hearings on the bill, see: U.S. Congress, House of Representatives, *Report to Accompany H.R. 15757, Health Manpower Act of 1968*, House Report No. 1634 (Washington, D.C.: Government Printing Office, 1968); U.S. Congress, House of Representatives, Committee on Interstate and Foreign Commerce, Subcommittee on Public Health and Welfare, *Health Manpower Act of 1968*, Hearings, 90th Cong., 2nd sess. (on H.R. 15757), 11, 12, 13 June (Washington, D.C.: Government Printing Office, 1968); and U.S. Congress, Senate, *Hearings Before the Subcommittee on Health of the Committee on Labor and Public Welfare, United States Senate, 90th Congress, 2nd sess.*, Hearings, 90th Cong., 2nd sess. (on S. 3095), 20–21 March (Washington, D.C.: Government Printing Office, 1968).

59   Kalisch and Kalisch, *Federal Influence*, p. 419.

60   Ibid., p. 424.

61   ANA, *Facts About Nursing* (1970–1971), p. 75.

62   Kalisch and Kalisch, *Federal Influence*, pp. 423–424.

63   Ibid., p. 426.

64   Ibid., p. 428.

65   Ibid., p. 420.

Chapter 7

1   W. K. Kellogg Foundation, "Annual Report of the Officers to the Members of the Foundation" (Battle Creek, Mich.: foundation archives, 1951–1952), p. 117; Philip A. Kalisch and Beatrice J. Kalisch, *The Advance of American Nursing*, 1st ed. (Boston: Little, Brown, 1978), p. 537.

2   Shirley H. Fondiller, *The Entry Dilemma: The National League for Nursing and the*

Higher Education Movement, 1952–1972, League Exchange No. 132 (New York: NLN, 1983), pp. 21, 28.

3   Unpublished overview by ANA of its action in nursing education (mimeographed), author's files.

4   Quoted in ibid., and by Fondiller, *Entry Dilemma*, p. 45.

5   Philip A. Kalisch and Beatrice J. Kalisch, *The Federal Influence and Impact on Nursing* (Hyattsville, Md.: U.S. Department of Health and Human Services, June 1980), p. 336.

6   Fondiller, *Entry Dilemma*, p. 45.

7   Ibid., pp. 45–50. Quotation on p. 46.

8   From the committee's report, entitled "This is the National League of Nursing," quoted in ibid., p. 46.

9   Mimeographed, in author's files.

10   Fondiller, *Entry Dilemma*, p. 41.

11   Ibid.

12   Ibid., pp. 41–42.

13   Ibid., p. 42.

14   Ibid.

15   "Opportunities for Education in Nursing" was first published by NLN in *Nursing Outlook* 8 (September 1980) and later under the title *Nursing Education Programs Today*.

16   Fondiller, *Entry Dilemma*, p. 30.

17   Ibid., p. 56.

18   NLN, Committee on Perspectives, *Perspectives for Nursing* (New York: NLN, 1965).

19   ANA, *Facts About Nursing* (1970–1971), p. 94.

20   *Perspectives for Nursing*, p. 21.

21   ANA report (mimeographed), author's files.

22   Ibid.

23   Kansas City, Mo.: American Nurses' Association, 1965. It was publication no. G-83, 17 pages long. The text was also published in the *American Journal of Nursing* in December 1965.

24   Quoted in ANA report (mimeographed), author's files.

25   Ibid.

26   Ibid.

27   ANA, *Position Paper*, pp. 14, 15.

28   ANA report (mimeographed), author's files.

29   Fondiller, *Entry Dilemma*, p. 55.

30   Percentages computed from numbers reported in ANA, *Facts About Nursing* (1970–1971), pp. 94, 81, 75.

31   ANA report (mimeographed), author's files.

32   Fondiller, *Entry Dilemma*, p. 59.

33   Ibid., pp. 59, 60.

34   Ibid., p. 60.

35   As quoted in ibid.

36   Ibid., pp. 103–104.

37   Ibid., p. 66.

38   Mildred L. Montag, "Looking Back: Associate Degree Education in Perspective," *Nursing Outlook* 28 (1980): 249.

39   A. R. Rines, "Associate Degree Nursing Education: History, Development, and Rationale," *Nursing Outlook* 25 (1977): 497.

40   Ruth Matheney, "Technical Nursing" (undated mimeographed report circulated by

NLN), author's files. See also R. V. Matheney, "A Definition of Technical Nursing," *Proceedings: Toward Differentiation of Baccalaureate and Associate Degree Nursing Education and Practice Workshop* (San Francisco: University of California, 1969).

41   Cited by Matheney in unpublished "Technical Nursing"; see also N. Harris, "Technical Education: Problem for the Present, Promise for the Future," *American Journal of Nursing* 63 (1963): 95–99, which defines and discusses the growing need for technical education in nursing.

42   ANA report (mimeographed), author's files.

43   Fondiller, *Entry Dilemma*, p. 55.

44   See "The American Nurses' Association and the National League for Nursing Joint Statement on Community Planning for Nursing Education," Appendix C of ibid., p. 121. The statement was issued in June 1966.

45   NLN, *Guidelines for Assessing the Nursing Education Needs of a Community*, Publication No. 11–1245 (New York: NLN, 1967).

46   Fondiller, *Entry Dilemma*, p. 66.

Chapter 8

1   ANA, *Facts About Nursing* (1970–1971), p. 91; (1980–1981), p. 152.

2   ANA, *Facts About Nursing* (1970–1971), p. 75.

3   B. L. Forest, "Utilization of Associate Degree Nursing Graduates in General Hospitals" (Ph.D. diss., Teachers College, Columbia University, 1968). The published version is *Utilization of Associate Degree Nursing Graduates in General Hospitals*, Publication No. 23–1290 (New York: NLN, 1968).

4   Robert E. Kinsinger, "The Crucial Role of Community College Administrators in the National Growth and Maintenance of Associate Degree Nursing Programs" (unpublished paper submitted to the author, 1986), p. 1.

5   See the companion volume to the present work, *Associate Degree Nursing Education: An Historical Annotated Bibliography* (city: publisher, year), for listing of examples.

6   Kenneth C. Green, "The Educational 'Pipeline' in Nursing," *Journal of Professional Nursing* July-August 1987, pp. 247–257.

7   ANA, *Facts About Nursing* (1980–1981), p. 152.

8   Kinsinger, "Crucial Role of Community College Administrators," pp. 1–2.

9   Barbara L. Tate and Elizabeth Carnegie, "Negro Admissions, Enrollments, and Graduations—1963," *Nursing Outlook* 13 (February 1965), as cited by Shirley H. Fondiller, *The Entry Dilemma: The National League for Nursing and the Higher Education Movement, 1952–1972*, League Exchange No. 132, NLN Publication No. 41–1896 (New York: NLN, 1983), p. 53.

10   Fondiller, *Entry Dilemma*, p. 52.

11   Ibid., p. 74.

12   Ibid., p. 81; ANA, *Facts About Nursing, 1970–1971*, pp. 94, 75.

13   Sylvia Lande, *A National Survey of Associate Degree Programs* (New York: NLN, 1969), as cited in Fondiller, *Entry Dilemma*, p. 81.

14   ANA, *Facts About Nursing* (1970–1971), p. 191, and (1980–1981), p. 267.

15   Unpublished overview by ANA of its action in nursing education (mimeographed), in author's files.

16   Mildred L. Montag, "Looking Back: Associate Degree Education in Perspective," *Nursing Outlook* 28 (1980): 249.

17   Rena E. Boyle et al., *Baccalaureate Education for the Registered Nurse Student*, Proceedings of conference of the Department of Baccalaureate and Higher Degree Pro-

grams, St. Louis, Mo. (New York: NLN, 1966).

18   Described in unpublished overview by ANA of its action in nursing education (mimeographed), in author's files.

19   University of California, *Proceedings: Toward Differentiation of Baccalaureate and Associate Degree Nursing Education and Practice Workshop* (San Francisco: University of California, 1969); Mary Searight, "The Second Step: A Baccalaureate Program for RNs," *California Nurse* 68, Suppl. NE4 (1971).

20   L. C. Dustan, "Needed: Articulation Between Nursing Education Programs and Institutions of Higher Learning," *Nursing Outlook* 18, no. 12 (1970): 34–37 (also available from NTIS); see also A. Schoenmaker, "An Articulated Nursing Program: Five Years Later," *Nursing Outlook* 23 (1975): 110–113.

21   Anon., "Now, an Associate Degree Without Attending College: A Career-Ladder Breakthrough," *RN* 35, no. 12 (1972): 50; see also E. B. Nyquist, "The Regents External Degrees," in NLN, *Associate Degree Education for Nursing—Current Issues, 1973* (New York: NLN, 1973), and idem, "The External Degree Program and Nursing," *Nursing Outlook* 21 (1973): 372–377.

22   Publication No. 15–1473 (1972); no longer available at NLN.

23   Fondiller, *Entry Dilemma*, p. 68. See also L. Y. Kelly, "Open Curriculum—What and Why?" *American Journal of Nursing* 74 (1974): 2232–2238.

24   J. P. Lysaught, *Action in Affirmation: Toward an Unambiguous Profession of Nursing* (New York: McGraw-Hill, 1981).

25   National Commission on Nursing, *Initial Report and Preliminary Recommendations* (Chicago: The Hospital Research and Education Trust, 1981); idem, *Summary Report and Recommendations* (Chicago: The Hospital Research and Education Trust, 1983). The commission's charge is described on p. xiii of the latter.

26   Institute of Medicine, Division of Health Care Services, *Nursing and Nursing Education: Public Policies and Private Actions* (Washington, D.C.: National Academy Press, 1983), p. xv.

27   Many of the recommendations by the three studies that were not directly related to basic nursing education are not discussed here, though they were to have great import to other sectors of the nursing community.

Chapter 9

1   U.S. Bureau of the Census, *Historical Statistics of the United States: Colonial Times to 1970* (Washington, D.C.: Government Printing Office, 1975), pt. 1, pp. 73–74 (tables B221–235 and B236–247).

2   ANA, *Facts About Nursing* (1974–75), p. 3; *Facts on File* (1968), p. 15.

3   Peter I. Buerhaus, "Not Just Another Nursing Shortage," *Nursing Economics* 5 (November-December 1987): p. 269 (table 1).

4   Kenneth C. Green, "The Educational 'Pipeline' in Nursing," *Journal of Professional Nursing*, July-August 1987, pp. 247–257.

5   Philip A. Kalisch and Beatrice J. Kalisch, *The Federal Influence and Impact on Nursing* (Hyattsville, Md.: U.S. Department of Health and Human Services, June 1980), p. 437.

6   For a summary of the efforts of the division to reduce the shortage of nurses, see U.S. Congress, Senate, Subcommittee on Departments of Labor and HEW Appropriations, *Departments of Labor and Health, Education, and Welfare and Related Agencies Appropriations, FY 72. Part 6: NIH*, Hearings, 92nd Cong., 1st sess., 20, 21 July (Washington, D.C.: Government Printing Office, 1971), pp. 4346–4355.

7 S. H. Altman, *Present and Future Supply of Registered Nurses*, DHEW Publication No. NIH 72–134 (Washington, D.C.: U.S. Public Health Service, Division of Nursing, 1971).

8 Kalisch and Kalisch, *Federal Influence*, pp. 452, 459, 460.

9 Ibid., pp. 460–464.

10 Ibid., p. 463.

11 Ibid., p. 482.

12 Ibid., pp. 470, 473.

13 See, for example, U.S. Congress, House of Representatives, Subcommittee on Public Health and Environment, *Health Professions Educational Assistance Amendments of 1971, Part 2*, Hearings, 92nd Cong., 1st sess. (Committee Serial No. 92–11), 21–23, 27–29 April (Washington, D.C.: Government Printing Office, 1971). The ANA testified in favor of expanded aid to meet nursing shortages and educational needs (pp. 747–758); the NLN agreed but focused on the needs of disadvantaged and minority students (pp. 773–778). The Association of Deans of College and University Schools of Nursing also appeared; it addressed issues of distribution of funds between diploma and ADN programs (pp. 802–812).

14 ANA summary report (mimeographed), author's files.

15 Kalisch and Kalisch, *Federal Influence*, p. 451 and passim.

16 Ibid., p. 483.

17 Ibid.

18 Ibid., p. 486.

19 Ibid., p. 497.

20 Ibid., p. 473.

21 Ibid., p. 485.

22 Ibid., pp. 488–502.

23 Ibid., p. 503. See also U.S. Congress, Senate, Subcommittee on Departments of Labor and Health, Education, and Welfare Appropriations, *Departments of Labor, and Health, Education, and Welfare, and Related Agencies Appropriations, FY 75, Part 3*, Hearings, 93rd Cong., 2nd sess. (on H.R. 15580), 14–16, 20, 22 May (Washington, D.C.: Government Printing Office, 1974), which includes the testimony of the director of the Division of Nursing to proposed cuts in the health manpower program.

24 Kalisch and Kalisch, *Federal Influence*, pp. 505–506, 503, and passim.

25 Ibid., p. 503.

26 Buerhaus, "Not Just Another Nursing Shortage," p. 269 (table 1).

27 Kalisch and Kalisch, *Federal Influence*, p. 509.

28 Buerhaus, "Nursing Shortage," p. 269.

29 Kalisch and Kalisch, *Federal Influence*, pp. 511–515.

30 Ibid., p. 517.

31 *Report on Nursing*, excerpted from *Fifth Report to the President and the Congress on the Status of Health Personnel in the United States, March 1986* and issued separately as NTIS Accession No. HRP 0906804 (Rockville, Md.: U.S. Department of Health and Human Services, 1986). See especially p. 10–56.

32 ANA overview of its action in education (mimeographed), in author's files.

33 ANA, *Facts About Nursing* (1970–1971), p. 94, and (1980–1981), p. 152.

34 In 1975 the ADN accounted for 44 percent, the diploma 29 percent, and the BSN 27 percent of all basic nursing programs. The baccalaureate had gained 11 percentage points since 1965. Ibid. (1980–1981), p. 152.

35 ANA overview (mimeographed), author's files.

36 Ibid.

37 Ibid.
38 Shirley H. Fondiller, *The Entry Dilemma: The National League for Nursing and the Higher Education Movement, 1952–1972*, League Exchange No. 132, NLN Publication No. 41–1896 (New York: NLN, 1983), p. 68; National League for Nursing, *Working Paper of the NLN Task Force on Competencies of Graduates of Nursing Programs*, Publication No. 14–1787 (New York: NLN, 1979; also available as NTIS No. HRP-0030576/3). See also the later version: NLN Task Force on Competencies of Graduates of Nursing Programs, *Competencies of Graduates of Nursing Programs*, Publication No. 14–1905 (New York: NLN, 1982).
39 "Statement on Nursing Roles—Scope and Preparation," Appendix G of Fondiller, *Entry Dilemma*, pp. 123–124.

Chapter 10

1 ANA, *Facts About Nursing* (1980–1981), p. 152.
2 Ibid., p. 133.
3 This account of the planning and development of the project is based on the author's own involvement, on records in her files, and the interim and final reports circulated among those who directed parts of the overall project. All formal reports are on file at the W. K. Kellogg Foundation, Battle Creek, Mich.
4 The detailed reports of the subprojects are on file at the W. K. Kellogg Foundation in Battle Creek, Mich. No attempt has been made here to provide comprehensive summaries of every one of them.
5 NLN, Council of Associate Degree Programs, *Competencies of the Associate Degree Nurse on Entry into Practice*, Publication No. 23–1731 (New York: NLN, 1978). Also published in *Nursing Outlook* 26 (1978): 457–458.
6 Mildred L. Montag, "Looking Back: Associate Degree Education in Perspective," *Nursing Outlook* 28 (1980): 248.
7 Eileen M. Williams and Marcia Scott-Warner, eds., *The Preparation and Utilization of New Nursing Graduates* (Boulder, Colo.: Western Interstate Commission for Higher Education, July 1985).

Chapter 11

1 ANA, *Facts About Nursing* (1970–1971), p. 94.
2 Data on file at the AAJC, 1986.
3 Report of survey by Thomas B. Merton (1964), Microfilm 159, W. K. Kellogg Foundation archives, Battle Creek, Mich.
4 Report of Conference on the Preparation of Instructors and Directors of ADN Programs (O'Hare Inn, Chicago, April 1965), Microfilm 159, W. K. Kellogg Foundation archives, Battle Creek, Mich.
5 W. K. Kellogg Foundation, "Associate Degree Programs in Nursing," in Nursing Division section of "Annual Program Reports to the Board of Trustees" (Battle Creek, Mich.: foundation archives, 19 September 1966), pp. 19–20.
6 W. K. Kellogg Foundation, "Associate Degree Nursing Programs" in Health Programs reports in "Annual Program Reports to the Board of Trustees" (Battle Creek, Mich.: foundation archives, 18 September 1967), pp. 22–23; "Demonstration Center" in ibid. (22 November 1968), pp. 19–20.
7 W. K. Kellogg Foundation, "Associate Degree in Nursing," in Nursing Division and General Programs report in "Annual Program Reports to the Board of Trustees" (Bat-

tle Creek, Mich.: foundation archives, 16 August 1960), pp. 8–9.

8   W. K. Kellogg Foundation, "Associate Degree Programs in Nursing," in Nursing Division report in "Annual Program Reports to the Board of Trustees" (Battle Creek, Mich.:
foundation archives, 19 September 1966), pp. 18–19; Anon., *Report of a Workshop
on Curriculum for Teachers in Associate Degree Nursing* (Memphis: University of
Tennessee College of Nursing, 1966).

9   W. K. Kellogg Foundation, "Graduate Education—United States," in Health Programs
report in "Annual Program Reports to the Board of Trustees" (Battle Creek, Mich.:
foundation archives, 18 September 1967), pp. 10–11.

10   W. K. Kellogg Foundation, "Faculty Preparation," in report on nursing projects in
"Annual Program Reports to the Board of Trustees" (Battle Creek, Mich.: foundation
archives, 1969–1970), pp. 11–12.

11   S. Rasmussen, Faculty Preparation and Professional Development for Associate Degree
Nursing Program: Summary Project Report to the W. K. Kellogg Foundation (Boston:
Boston University School of Nursing, 1970), Microfilm 159, W. K. Kellogg Founda-
tion archives, Battle Creek, Mich.

12   W. K. Kellogg Foundation, "Faculty Preparation," in nursing project reports in "Annual
Program Reports to the Board of Trustees" (Battle Creek, Mich.: foundation archives,
1969–1970), pp. 14–15; "Associate Degree Programs" in ibid. (1970–1971), p. 14.

13   W. K. Kellogg Foundation, "Associate Degree Programs," in nursing project reports in
"Annual Program Reports to the Board of Trustees" (Battle Creek, Mich.: foundation
archives, 1970–1971), p. 13.

14   The account in this chapter of the work at the various sites is based on the author's
own involvement, on records in her files, and on the progress and final reports circulated among those who directed parts of the overall project. All formal project reports
are on file at the W. K. Kellogg Foundation, Battle Creek, Mich. No attempt is made
here to report comprehensively the work and findings at each site.

Chapter 12

1   ANA, *Facts About Nursing* (1986–1987), p. 42, reports 42,372 ADN graduates of a
total of 78,474; [Sally Solomon], *Nursing Data Review, 1985*, Publication No. 19–1994
(New York: NLN, Division of Public Policy and Research, 1986), p. 35, reports 41,849
from a total of 77,408.

2   American Hospital Association, "Preliminary Report to Respondents: Hospital Nursing Personnel Survey—1985 American Hospital Association," August 1986, p. 5
(mimeographed).

3   *Legislative Network for Nurses* 5 (31 May 1988): 2, quoting statistics reported in
AHA News, 16 May 1988.

4   Claire M. Fagin, "The Visible Problems of an 'Invisible' Profession: The Crisis and
Challenge for Nursing," *Inquiry* 24 (Summer 1987): 121.

5   As reported in the *Chronicle of Higher Education*, 1 April 1987, p. 28.

6   *Health Professions Report* 17 (20 June 1988): 4.

7   Ibid., p. 3.

8   Kenneth C. Green, "The Educational 'Pipeline' in Nursing," *Journal of Professional
Nursing*, July-August 1987, p. 251. Dr. Green's article was the keynote speech at the
March 1987 meeting of AACN.

9   Sharon Johnson, "The Nursing Profession Is in Need of Care," *New York Times*, 22
March 1987.

10   *Health Professions Report* 17 (20 June 1988): 4.

11 Ibid., p. 4.

12 Computed from data in ANA, *Facts About Nursing* (1970–1971, 1980–1981, 1984–1985).

13 For a discussion of the issues, see, e.g., Mary E. Foley, "The Politics of Collective Bargaining," in Diana J. Mason and Susan W. Talbott, eds., *Political Action Handbook for Nurses: Changing the Workplace, Government, Organizations, and Community* (Menlo Park, Calif.: Addison-Wesley, 1985), pp. 265–282; Norma L. McKay and Walter A. Lumley, "Nonunionized Collective Action: The Staff Nurse Forum," in ibid., pp. 286–291. For recent statistics on unionization, see Karen Southwich, "Snags Delay Unionizing Efforts," *Healthweek*, 28 November 1988, pp. 1, 35.

14 ANA, *Capital Update* 6 (10 June 1988): 2.

15 FNHP President Candice Owley, as quoted in *Health Professions Report* 17 (6 June 1988): 2.

16 Ibid., pp. 2–3.

17 "Strategy Document on Short-Term Strategies to Resolve the Nursing Shortage," endorsed by thirty-four nursing organizations at a meeting hosted by the Tri Council on 5 May 1988, and circulated by the AACN to its members on 17 May 1988.

18 For details, see ANA *Capital Update* 6 (27 May 1988): 2, 5; AACN *Newsletter* 14 (June 1988): 1–2.

19 Pamela J. Maraldo, "Executive Director Wire" (NLN), August 1987, p. 1.

20 See, e.g., "Differentiated Practice: The Cornerstone of Nursing's Future," transcript of Forum No. 5, NCNP 1987 Invitational Conference, San Diego, Calif., 5–6 November 1987 (mimeographed).

21 [Solomon], *Nursing Data Review, 1985*, p. 43.

22 Fagin, "Visible Problems," p. 120.

Bibliography

Consultants

Virginia Allen, Middlesex County College, Edison, New Jersey

Margaret Applegate, Indiana University, Indianapolis, Indiana

Georgeen Harriet DeChow, retired (Manatee Junior College, Bradenton, Florida)

Helen K. Grace, W. K. Kellogg Foundation

Robert E. Kinsinger, retired (W. K. Kellogg Foundation)

Mildred L. Montag, retired (Director, Cooperative Research Project)

Marilyn Schalit, Higher Education Research Institute, UCLA

Verle Waters, Ohlone College School of Nursing, Fremont, California

W. K. Kellogg Foundation Archives

W. K. Kellogg Foundation. "Annual Program Reports to the Board of Trustees." Battle Creek, Mich.: foundation archives, 1958–.

W. K. Kellogg Foundation. "Annual Report of the Officers of the W. K. Kellogg Foundation to the Members of the Foundation." Battle Creek, Mich.: foundation archives, 1947–.

W. K. Kellogg Foundation. "Bimonthly Reports of the Officers to the Board of Trustees." Battle Creek, Mich.: foundation archives, 1949–.

Merton, Thomas B. Report of survey. Microfilm 159. Battle Creek, Mich.: foundation archives, 1964.

Rasmussen, S. Faculty Preparation and Professional Development for Associate Degree Nursing Program: Summary Project Report to the W. K. Kellogg Foundation. Boston: Boston University School of Nursing, 1970. (Also available on Microfilm 159. Battle Creek, Mich.: foundation archives.)

Report of Conference on the Preparation of Instructors and Directors of ADN Programs (O'Hare Inn, Chicago, April 1965). Microfilm 159. Battle Creek, Mich.: W. K. Kellogg Foundation archives.

Government Documents

Altman, S. H. Present and Future Supply of Registered Nurses. DHEW Publication No. NIH 72-134. Washington, D.C.: U.S. Public Health Service, Division of Nursing, 1971.

Bureau of the Health Professions. *Report on Nursing*, excerpted from *Fifth Report to the President and the Congress on the Status of Health Personnel in the United States, March 1986*, and issued separately as NTIS Accession No. HRP 0906804. Rockville, Md.: U.S. Department of Health and Human Services, 1986.

Ewing, O. R. *The Nation's Health: A Report to the President*. Washington, D.C.: Government Printing Office, 1948.

Kalisch, Philip A., and Kalisch, Beatrice J. *The Federal Influence and Impact on Nursing*. Hyattsville, Md.: U.S. Department of Health and Human Services, June 1980.

President's Commission on Higher Education. *Establishing the Goals*. 2 vols. Washington, D.C.: Government Printing Office, 1967.

Report of the National Advisory Commission on Health Manpower. Washington, D.C.: Government Printing Office, 1967.

United States. An Act to Amend the Public Health Service Act to Extend and Improve the Programs Related to the Training of Nurses . . . (Public Law 90–490). *Statutes at Large* 82 (1968): 773–789.

United States. An Act to Amend the Public Health Service Act to Increase the Opportunities for Professional Nursing Personnel, and for Other Purposes (Public Law 88–581). *Statutes at Large* 78 (1964): 908–919.

U.S. Bureau of the Census. *Historical Statistics of the United States: Colonial Times to 1970*. Washington, D.C.: Government Printing Office, 1975.

U.S. Bureau of the Census. *Statistical Abstract of the United States*. 105th ed. Washington, D.C.: Government Printing Office, 1984.

U.S. Bureau of the Census. *Statistical Abstract of the United States*, 107th ed. Washington, D.C.: Government Printing Office, 1987.

U.S. Bureau of Labor Statistics. *The Economic Status of Registered Professional Nurses, 1946–47*. Bulletin No. 931. Washington, D.C.: Government Printing Office, 1947.

U.S. Congress, House of Representatives. *Hearings Before a Subcommittee of the Committee on Interstate & Foreign Commerce, House of Representatives—Health Amendments Act of 1956 (Nurse and Public Health Personnel Training—Commission on Nursing Services)*. Hearings, 84th Cong., 2nd sess. (on H.R. 11549), 13, 14, 15 June. Washington, D.C.: Government Printing Office, 1956.

U.S. Congress, House of Representatives. *Report to Accompany H.R. 15757, Health Manpower Act of 1968*. House Report No. 1634. Washington, D.C.: Government Printing Office, 1968.

U.S. Congress, House of Representatives, Committee on Interstate and Foreign Commerce, Subcommittee on Public Health and Safety. *Nurse Training Act of 1964*. Hearings, 88th Cong., 2nd sess., 8–10 April. Washington, D.C.: Government Printing Office, 1964.

U.S. Congress, House of Representatives, Committee on Interstate and Foreign Commerce, Subcommittee on Public Health and Welfare. *Health Manpower Act of 1968*. Hearings, 90th Cong., 2nd sess. (on H.R. 15757), 11, 12, 13 June. Washington, D.C.: Government Printing Office, 1968.

U.S. Congress, House of Representatives, Subcommittee on Public Health and Environment. *Health Professions Educational Assistance Amendments of 1971, Part 2*. Hearings, 92nd Cong., 1st sess. (Committee Serial No. 92-11), 21–23, 27–29 April. Washington, D.C.: Government Printing Office, 1971.

U.S. Congress, Senate. *Hearings Before the Subcommittee on Health of the Committee on Labor and Public Welfare, United States Senate, 90th Congress, 2nd sess.* Hearings, 90th Cong., 2nd sess. (on S. 2095), 20–21 March. Washington, D.C.: Government Printing Office, 1968.

U.S. Congress, Senate, Committee on Labor and Public Welfare. *Nurse Training Act of 1964*. Senate Report No. 88-1378. Washington, D.C.: Government Printing Office, 1964.

U.S. Congress, Senate, Subcommittee on Departments of Labor and Health, Education, and Welfare appropriations. *Departments of Labor, and Health, Education, and Welfare, and Related Agencies Appropriations, FY 75, Part 3*. Hearings, 93rd Cong., 2nd sess. (on H.R. 15580), 14–16, 20, 22 May. Washington, D.C.: Government Printing Office, 1974.

U.S. Congress, Senate, Subcommittee on Departments of Labor and HEW Appropriations. *Departments of Labor and Health, Education, and Welfare and Related Agencies Appropriations, FY 72. Part 6: NIH*. Hearings, 92nd Cong., 1st sess., 20, 21 July. Washington, D.C.: Government Printing Office, 1971.

U.S. DHEW. *Nurse Training Act of 1964: Program Review Report*. PHS Publication No. 1740. Washington, D.C.: Government Printing Office, December 1967.

U.S. DHEW. *The Nurse Training Act of 1964*. PHS Publication No. 1154. Washington, D.C.: Government Printing Office, 1965. Other pamphlets in this series: *Professional Nurse Traineeship Program*. PHS Publication No. 1154-1; *Project Grants for Improvements in Nurse Training*. PHS Publication No. 1154-2; *Payments to Diploma Schools of Nursing*. PHS Publication No. 1154-3; *Nursing Student Loan Program: Information for Schools*. PHS Publication No. 1154-4; *Construction Grants Program for Schools of Nursing*. PHS Publication No. 1154-5. Updates published in 1969.

U.S. DHEW, Office of the Surgeon General. *Toward Quality in Nursing: Needs and Goals*. PHS Publication No. 992. Washington, D.C.: Government Printing Office, 1963.

U.S. DHEW, Public Health Service. *Nursing Education Facilities, Programing Considerations and Architectural Guide: Report of the Joint Committee on Educational Facilities for Nursing of the National League for Nursing and the Public Health Service*. PHS Publication No. 1180-F-1B. Washington, D.C.: Government Printing Office, 1964.

Nursing Organization Publications

American Association of Colleges of Nursing. *Newsletter*. 1987–1988.

ANA. *Capital Update* [newsletter] 6 (27 May and 10 June 1988).

ANA. *Facts About Nursing*. 1946 through 1986–1987.

ANA. *A Position Paper on Educational Preparation for Nurse Practitioners and Assistants to Nurses*. Publication No. G-83. Kansas City, Mo.: author, 1965. Also published in the *American Journal of Nursing*, December 1965.

Boyle, Rena E., et al. *Baccalaureate Education for the Registered Nurse Student*. Proceedings of conference of the Department of Baccalaureate and Higher Degree Programs, St. Louis, Mo. New York: NLN, 1966.

Fondiller, Shirley H. *The Entry Dilemma: The National League for Nursing and the Higher Education Movement, 1952–1972*. League Exchange No. 132, NLN Publication No. 41-1896. New York: NLN, 1983.

Forest, B. L. *Utilization of Associate Degree Nursing Graduates in General Hospitals*. Publication No. 23-1290. New York: NLN, 1968. Also Ph.D. diss., Teachers College, Columbia University, 1968.

Lande, Sylvia. *A National Survey of Associate Degree Programs*. New York: NLN, 1969.

Maraldo, Pamela J. "Executive Director Wire." August 1987.

Matheney, Ruth. "Technical Nursing." Undated mimeographed report circulated by NLN; author's files.

NLN. *The Associate Degree Program—A Step to the Baccalaureate Degree in Nursing*.

Publication No. 15-1473. New York: author, 1972. No longer available at NLN.

NLN. *Guidelines for Assessing the Nursing Education Needs of a Community.* Publication No. 11-1245. New York: author, 1967.

NLN. *Leadership for Quality* (report of a conference held by the Department of Associate Degree Programs, St. Louis, March 1966). Publication No. 12-1240. New York: author, 1966.

NLN. *Working Paper of the NLN Task Force on Competencies of Graduates of Nursing Programs.* Publication No. 14-1787. New York: author, 1979. Also available as NTIS No. HRP-0030576/3.

NLN, Committee on Perspectives. *Perspectives for Nursing.* New York: author, 1965.

NLN, Council of Associate Degree Programs. *Competencies of the Associate Degree Nurse on Entry into Practice.* Pub. No. 23-1731. New York: author, 1978. Also published in *Nursing Outlook* 26 (1978): 457–458.

NLN, Department of Diploma and Associate Degree Programs. *Planning for Nursing Education in a Community College.* League Exchange No. 32, Publication No. 16-703. New York: author, 1958.

NLN Task Force on Competencies of Graduates of Nursing Programs. *Competencies of Graduates of Nursing Programs.* Publication No. 14-1905. New York: author, 1982.

Nyquist, E. B. "The Regents External Degrees." In NLN, *Associate Degree Education for Nursing—Current Issues, 1973.* New York: author, 1973.

[Solomon, Sally.] *Nursing Data Review, 1985.* Publication No. 19-1994. New York: NLN, Division of Public Policy and Research, 1986.

Monographs and Books

Abdellah, Faye G., Beland, Irene L., Martin, Alameda, and Matheney, Ruth V. *Patient-Centered Approaches to Nursing.* New York: Macmillan, 1961.

Anderson, Bernice. *Nursing Education in Community Junior Colleges: A Four-State 5-Year Experience in the Development of Associate Degree Programs.* Philadelphia: J. B. Lippincott, 1966.

Anonymous. *Report of a Workshop on Curriculum for Teachers in Associate Degree Nursing.* Memphis: University of Tennessee College of Nursing, 1966.

Ashley, Jo Ann. *Hospitals, Paternalism, and the Role of the Nurse.* New York: Teachers College Press, Columbia University, 1976.

Astin, Alexander W. *American Freshmen: National Norms, Fall 1987.* Los Angeles: Higher Education Research Institute, UCLA, 1987.

Astin, Alexander W. *American Freshmen: Twenty-Year Trends.* Los Angeles: Higher Education Research Institute, UCLA, 1987.

Bloom, Benjamin S. *Taxonomy of Education Objectives: Handbook I, Cognitive Domain.* New York: David McKay, 1956.

Bogue, Jesse Parker. *The Community College.* New York: McGraw-Hill, 1950.

Brown, E. L. *Nursing for the Future: A Report Prepared for the National Nursing Council.* New York: Russell Sage Foundation, 1948.

California, University of. *Proceedings: Toward a Differentiation of Baccalaureate and Associate Degree Nursing Education and Practice Workshop.* San Francisco: author, 1969.

Campion, Frank D. *The AMA and U.S. Health Policy Since 1940.* Chicago: Chicago Review Press, 1984.

Commission on Hospital Care. *Hospital Care in the United States: A Study of the Function of the General Hospital, Its Role in the Care of All Types of Illness, and the*

Conduct of Activities Related to Patient Service, with Recommendations for Its Extension and Integration for More Adequate Care of the American Public. New York: Commonwealth Fund, 1947.

Diener, Thomas. *Growth of an American Invention: A Documentary History of the Junior and Community College Movement.* New York: Greenwood, 1986.

Edwards, Newton, and Richey, Herman G. *The School in the American Social Order.* 2nd ed. Boston: Houghton Mifflin, 1963.

Eells, W. C. "Historical Development: California." In *The Junior College.* Boston: Houghton Mifflin, 1931.

Fields, Ralph R. *The Community College Movement.* New York: McGraw-Hill, 1962.

Florida Community College Council. *The Community Junior College in Florida's Future: Report to the State Board of Education.* Tallahassee: Florida State Board of Education, 1957.

Fretwell, Elbert K., Jr. *Founding Public Junior Colleges.* New York: Teachers College, Columbia University, 1954.

Ginzberg, Eli. *A Program for the Nursing Profession.* New York: Macmillan, 1948.

Griffin, Gerald J., Kinsinger, Robert E., and Pitman, Avis J. *Clinical Nursing Instruction by Television.* New York: Teachers College, Columbia University, 1965.

Haase, Patricia T. (compiler). *Associate Degree Nursing Education: An Historical Annotated Bibliography, 1942–1983.* [to be updated].

Institute of Medicine, Division of Health Care Services. *Nursing and Nursing Education: Public Policies and Private Actions.* Washington, D.C.: National Academy Press, 1983.

Kalisch, Philip A., and Kalisch, Beatrice J. *The Advance of American Nursing.* 1st ed. Boston: Little, Brown, 1978. 2nd ed., 1986.

Lenburg, Carrie B. *The Clinical Performance Examination.* New York: Appleton-Century-Crofts, 1979.

Lysaught, J. P. *Action in Affirmation: Toward an Unambiguous Profession of Nursing.* New York: McGraw-Hill, 1981.

Mager, Robert F. *Preparing Educational Objectives.* Belmont, Calif.: Fearon Publishers, 1962.

Matheney, R. V., Nolan, B., Griffin, G. J., Griffin, J., and Ehrhart, A. *Fundamentals of Patient-Centered Nursing.* St. Louis: Mosby, 1964.

Monroe, Charles R. *Profile of the Community College: A Handbook.* San Francisco: Jossey-Bass, 1972.

National Commission on Nursing. *Initial Report and Preliminary Recommendations.* Chicago: The Hospital Research and Education Trust, 1981.

National Commission on Nursing. *Summary Report and Recommendations.* Chicago: The Hospital Research and Education Trust, 1983.

[New York] Nurse Resource Study Group, University of the State of New York. *Needs and Facilities in Professional Nursing Education.* Albany, N.Y.: author, 1959.

Postlethwait, Samuel N. *An Integrated Approach to Learning.* Edina, Minn.: Burgess, 1964.

Seedor, Marie M. *Programmed Instruction for Nursing in the Community College.* New York: Teachers College, Columbia University, 1963.

Thomas, Lewis. *The Medusa and the Snail.* New York: Bantam Books, 1980.

Tyler, Ralph W. *Basic Principles of Curriculum and Instruction.* Chicago: University of Chicago Press, 1949.

West, M., and Hawkins, C. *Nursing Schools at the Mid-Century.* New York: National Committee for the Improvement of Nursing Services, 1950.

Williams, Eileen M., and Scott-Warner, Marcia, eds. *The Preparation and Utilization of New Nursing Graduates.* Boulder, Colo.: Western Interstate Commission for Higher Education, July 1985.

Yett, Donald D. *An Economic Analysis of the Nurse Shortage.* Lexington, Mass.: Lexington Books, 1975.

Articles and Periodicals

Allen, Virginia O. "Pioneering Curricular Innovations Contributed by Associate Degree Nursing Educators." Unpublished paper submitted to the author, 1986.

Anonymous. "Now, an Associate Degree Without Attending College: A Career-Ladder Breakthrough." *RN* 35, no. 12 (1972): 50.

Bolton, Francis P. "Crisis in Health Care: Report to Congress on the Nursing Shortage." *Hospital* 28 (April 1954): 83–85.

Buerhaus, Peter I. "Not Just Another Nursing Shortage." *Nursing Economics* 5 (November-December 1987): 267–279.

Chronicle of Higher Education. 1987–1988.

DeChow, G. H. "The Development of an Associate Degree Nursing Program." *Journal of Nursing Education* 1 (September 1962): 9–10, 33–36.

"Differentiated Practice: The Cornerstone of Nursing's Future." Transcript of Forum No. 5, NCNP 1987 Invitational Conference, San Diego, Calif., 5–6 November 1987. Mimeograph.

Dustan, L. C. "Needed: Articulation Between Nursing Education Programs and Institutions of Higher Learning." *Nursing Outlook* 18, no. 12 (1970): 34–37. Also available from NTIS.

Fagin, Claire M. "The Visible Problems of an 'Invisible' Profession: The Crisis and Challenge for Nursing." *Inquiry* 24 (Summer 1987): 121.

Flanagan, John C. "The Critical Incident Technique." *Psychological Bulletin* 51 (1954): 327–358.

Foley, Mary E. "The Politics of Collective Bargaining." In Diana J. Mason and Susan W. Talbott, eds., *Political Action Handbook for Nurses: Changing the Workplace, Government, Organizations, and Community,* pp. 265–282. Menlo Park, Calif.: Addison-Wesley, 1985.

Galeener, J. T. "Group or Multiple Student Assignment." *Journal of Nursing Education* 5 (April 1966): 29–31.

Goodrich, A. W. "Nursing and National Defense." *American Journal of Nursing* 42 (1942): 11–16.

Green, Kenneth C. "The Educational 'Pipeline' in Nursing." *Journal of Professional Nursing,* July-August 1987, pp. 247–257.

Hardy, Mary Anderson. "The American Nurses' Association Influence on Federal Funding for Nursing Education, 1941–1984. *Nursing Research* 36, no. 1 (January-February 1987): 31–35.

Harris, N. "Technical Education: Problem for the Present, Promise for the Future." *American Journal of Nursing* 63 (1963): 95–99.

Haupt, A. C. "Our War Nursing Program." *American Journal of Nursing* 42 (1942): 1381–1385.

Health Professions Report. 1987–1988.

Johnson, Sharon. "The Nursing Profession Is in Need of Care." *New York Times,* 22 March 1987.

Kelly, L. Y. "Open Curriculum—What and Why?" *American Journal of Nursing* 74 (1974):

2232–2238.

Kinsinger, Robert E. "The Crucial Role of Community College Administrators in the National Growth and Maintenance of Associate Degree Nursing Programs." Unpublished paper submitted to the author, 1986.

Legislative Network for Nurses. 1988.

Lindsay, Frank B. "California Junior Colleges: Past and Present." *California Journal of Secondary Education* 22 (March 1947): 137–142.

McKay, Norma L., and Lumley, Walter A. "Nonunionized Collective Action: The Staff Nurse Forum." In Diana J. Mason and Susan W. Talbott, eds., *Political Action Handbook for Nurses: Changing the Workplace, Government, Organizations, and Community,* pp. 286–291. Menlo Park, Calif.: Addison-Wesley, 1985.

Matheney, R[uth] V. "A definition of Technical Nursing." In *Proceedings: Toward Differentiation of Baccalaureate and Associate Degree Nursing Education and Practice Workshop.* San Francisco: University of California, 1969.

Matheney, Ruth V. "Pre- and Post-Conference for Students." *American Journal of Nursing* 69 (1969): 286–289.

Montag, Mildred. "The Associate Degree Nursing Program." Unpublished paper submitted to the author, 1986.

Montag, Mildred L. "Looking Back: Associate Degree Education in Perspective." *Nursing Outlook* 28 (1980): 249.

NLN. "Opportunities for Education in Nursing." *Nursing Outlook* 8 (September 1980). Later published as *Nursing Education Programs Today.*

Nyquist, E. B. "The External Degree Program and Nursing." *Nursing Outlook* 21 (1973): 372–377.

Petry, Lucile. "How to Qualify Under the Act." *Modern Hospital* 61, no. 3 (1943): 60–61.

Petry, Lucile. "A Summing Up: The U.S. Cadet Nurse Corps." *American Journal of Nursing* 45 (1945): 1027–1028.

Petry, L., Arnstein, M., and Gillan, R. "Surveys Measure Nursing Resources." *American Journal of Nursing* 49 (1949): 770–772.

"Residency Training of Physician Veterans." *JAMA* 131 (1946): 1356.

Rines, Alice R. "Associate Degree Nursing Education: History, Development and Rationale." *Nursing Outlook* 25 (1977): 496–501.

Schoenmaker, A. "An Articulated Nursing Program: Five Years Later." *Nursing Outlook* 23 (1975): 110–113.

Searight, Mary. "The Second Step: A Baccalaureate Program for RNs." *California Nurse* 68, Suppl. NE4, 1971.

Simpson, June. "The Walk-Around Laboratory Practical Examination in Evaluating Clinical Nursing Skills." *Journal of Nursing Education* 6 (1967): 23–26.

Southwich, Karen. "Snags Delay Unionizing Efforts." *Healthweek,* 28 November 1988, pp. 1, 35.

Tate, Barbara L., and Carnegie, Elizabeth. "Negro Admissions, Enrollments, and Graduations—1963." *Nursing Outlook* 13 (February 1965).

Wattenbarger, J. L. "Florida's Community Junior Colleges and Nursing Education." *Florida Nurse* 10, no. 1 (1962): 35–36.

Index